Anti-Inflammatory Cookbook

50 Quick and Easy Recipes to Reduce Inflammation, Heal the Immune System, and Improve Overall Health

(7-Day Meal Plan to Help People Create Results, Starting from Their First Day!)

Clarissa Fleming

Table of Contents

Introduction

Chronic inflammation is a difficult and painful condition. What begins as a minor inconvenience can develop into more serious health concerns as time goes on until inflammation is interfering with your ability to complete tasks and enjoy activities. If you experience frequent joint pain, stiffness, redness, and swelling, you may be experiencing chronic inflammation. It can also manifest as an upset stomach and pain in the intestines and has been linked to health concerns like arthritis, type 2 diabetes, and certain types of cancers.

Despite the difficulties of living life with inflammation, it is possible to lessen symptoms and reduce how often inflammation occurs. Changes you make to your daily behaviors and lifestyle can have a dramatic effect on how often inflammation is able to slow you down. Alongside factors like exercise and pain management, your diet is one of the most effective ways to combat inflammation. Cutting out inflammatory foods and replacing them with fresh, whole ingredients can have a positive impact on your body and overall health. Best of all, you don't have to be a professional chef to follow these recipes.

This book contains 50 recipes that follow the plan set out by the anti-inflammatory diet for reducing inflamed tissue and managing symptoms of pain and discomfort. Using these easy, quick, and simple recipes, you can improve your health and ease your suffering from the comfort of your own kitchen.

What Is an Anti-Inflammatory Diet?

An anti-inflammatory diet aims to reduce inflammation by altering the kinds of food you eat. This means cutting out pro-inflammatory foods, but it also means trying new and exciting recipes full of ingredients that taste great and are great for you. Anti-inflammatory diets have recently risen in popularity to combat the high-sugar and high-carb foods that have become common staples of our diets even though these foods are unhealthy and can lead to health complications in the long run. The diet is especially beneficial to reduce symptoms from cases of chronic inflammation that are otherwise persistent and painful, but it can also be used as a guideline for reducing your intake of sugars, processed meals, and saturated and trans fats.

The following chapters provide background information on inflammation as a process of the body, as well as ways to combat chronic inflammation. You will learn what foods to avoid and what foods to add to your diet to keep yourself happy, healthy, and of course, full. The 50 recipes that follow make use of these beneficial ingredients to craft delicious meals with minimal effort that are sure to reduce inflammation and pain.

Chapter 1: What Is Inflammation?

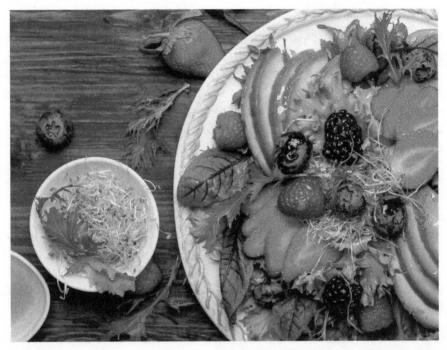

Inflammation is part of the body's automatic response to injuries and illnesses. It helps your body to target areas in need of attention by identifying the location of the damage or infection. It can result in redness and swelling in a certain area as the body tissues become inflamed. Your immune system uses white blood cells to attack anything it deems as harmful in an attempt to protect you. When your body's immune system is functioning properly, inflammation can help you heal from cuts or fight off an illness; when your immune system malfunctions, however, it can lead to excessive inflammation, swelling, and long-term pain.

Inflammation's Effects

Inflammation is not inherently good or bad. The same redness and swelling that occurs as an appropriate reaction to isolated incidents can worsen and develop into frequent pain and more serious health problems. If your body is functioning as it should, inflammation generally benefits you, but if your body is no longer able to differentiate harmful foreign invaders from your own cells, it can harm you instead.

There are two different types of inflammation, identified by how long the inflammation lasts and how much of the body it targets. Acute inflammation is a short-term condition that is highly focused on a small specific region of the body. You experience acute inflammation when you get a sore throat or when you bump your elbow. It is generally not a cause for concern, as it does not last for long and typically helps you recover from pain and sickness.

Chronic inflammation, on the other hand, can be a more painful and harmful condition. It is a more long-term response of your immune system, and it is often widespread throughout the body rather than targeting a specific area. Chronic inflammation is linked to the development of many different diseases, including heart problems, cancers, and digestive irregularities.

When Inflammation Is Helpful

Under normal circumstances, inflammation is an important part of your immune system. The regular function of inflammation is "a local response to cellular injury [...] which serves to initiate the elimination of toxic agents and the repair of damaged tissue" (Minihane et al., 2015, para. 2). It helps you combat viral and bacterial infections. It also assists in repairing injuries caused by cuts, bumps, and bruises. Without inflammation, your white blood cells would not know where to go in your body, and you would not be able to effectively fight off getting sick or quickly heal from a minor injury. While inflammation is a natural process of the body, your body's immune system does not always work as intended, which is when inflammation becomes chronic and painful.

When Inflammation Is Harmful

Long-lasting and persistently recurrent inflammation is a result of a malfunctioning and overactive immune system. Your body may flag a perfectly healthy area as one in need of repair, inflaming the area as white blood cells build up. This can become an autoimmune disorder, where your white blood cells begin to see your body's own cells as dangerous and attack the healthy cells. The occurrence of these cases can be attributed to a few different factors, one of which is the food you eat. "While there are genetic causes, the most important factor is believed to be the standard American diet, rich in pro-inflammatory compounds," as well as "lacking antioxidants and other nutrients that help and control inflammation". Diets high in inflammatory compounds worsen the frequency of inflammation and can contribute to the development of a variety of diseases.

Health Conditions Related to Inflammation

Many health conditions have been linked to high rates of inflammation and the resulting autoimmune disorders. Researchers have found that common human pathologies, such as atherosclerosis (plaque and fat build-up within arteries), neurodegenerative diseases like Parkinson's and Alzheimer's, and cancer (the most common human pathologies), are driven by the inflammatory process (Tomasi, Özben, and Skulachev, 2003, pg. v). These diseases can cause lifelong health complications if left untreated and should be addressed as soon as possible.

Heart Diseases

Chronic inflammation is a big component of heart diseases. Alongside high blood pressure and cholesterol, it is one of the leading contributors to health issues involving the heart. The heart muscles themselves can become inflamed, resulting in persistent symptoms of chest pain, shortness of breath, fatigue, and swelling of hands and feet. Inflammation can lead to clogged arteries and issues with blood flow, which can manifest in narrowed blood vessels and weakened pumping of blood. Chronic inflammation also increases your risk of serious, dangerous conditions like heart attacks and strokes because of these interruptions in blood flow. Lessening inflammation can help lower your chances of developing these serious, life-threatening issues.

Bowel Diseases

Digestive irregularities can range from inconvenient to actively dangerous, and any manifestation of digestive irregularities should be taken seriously. The main bowel diseases related to inflammation involve an inflamed digestive tract and are referred to under the umbrella term *inflammatory bowel disease* (IBD). Symptoms tend to fluctuate in severity and occur in waves. You may experience irregular bowel movements, fatigue, cramping, and fever. The two most frequently encountered types of IBD are ulcerative colitis and Crohn's disease. Ulcerative colitis involves sores and long-term inflammation in the large intestine, while Crohn's disease mainly affects the lining of the digestive tract and nearby tissues. Either condition can cause disruptions in daily life and can lead to potentially fatal complications if inflammation is not dealt with.

Arthritis

An overactive immune system can lead to painful joint inflammation characteristic of arthritis. This autoimmune disorder causes stiffness and swelling when moving joints, limiting your range of motion. Unlike osteoarthritis, which is caused by years of use and primarily appears later in life, forms of arthritis caused by inflammation can develop much earlier. There are a few varieties of arthritis that fall under this subheading. One of the most common is rheumatoid arthritis, which is typically widespread throughout the body and affects many joints at once. It also tends to heavily affect large, weight-bearing joints, such as the knee and hip.

In contrast, psoriatic arthritis tends to affect smaller joints, such as the fingers and toes, though it can also be present in large joints. It is accompanied by psoriasis, which is a skin condition involving patches of rough, scaly skin that is often reddened. Another form of inflammatory arthritis is gout. It is commonly associated with pain in the foot, especially the big toe. Gout is caused by chemicals released when breaking down certain foods and can best be eased by altering your diet.

Lupus

Lupus is a form of autoimmune disease that can produce symptoms of joint pain, fatigue, chest or abdominal pain, rashes, and severe headaches. It most commonly affects the whole body, though symptoms initially appear in an isolated area and spread over time. Lupus can also be worsened through exposure to the sun, requiring you to change lifestyle patterns and take extra precautions throughout the day to limit sunlight. The inflammation and autoimmune complications that lupus produces can severely affect a person's quality of life if no adjustments are made.

Inflammation that occurs in the thyroid gland is known as thyroiditis. It is an autoimmune condition in which your body attacks and inflames your own cells, localized on the thyroid gland. Your thyroid controls the hormones that govern your body's ability to metabolize food. Irregularities within the thyroid disrupt your metabolism and can cause notable impacts throughout the body. Inflammation initially causes your thyroid to release more hormones than normal. Once this occurs for an extended period of time, usually multiple weeks at once, your body's ability to produce the appropriate hormones can be weakened, leading to fewer metabolic hormones than usual being released. These two states may eventually stabilize for a period of time, but inflammation begins the cycle anew. This can lead to the development of two separate thyroid conditions: hypothyroidism and hyperthyroidism.

When your thyroid overproduces hormones, you can experience hyperthyroidism. This condition kicks your metabolism into high gear, past the normal functionality of your body. It can lead to extreme and unintentional weight loss, a rapid or irregular heartbeat, mood alterations, and trouble sleeping. You may feel hot more often than before, even in moderate temperatures. You may also develop pain and swelling in your throat around the thyroid as a result of the inflammation and over-activity.

Hypothyroidism, on the other hand, is characterized by a severe decrease in metabolic hormones being produced by your thyroid. Overproduction can wear out your body's ability to make hormones over time and leave you with a hormone deficiency. Its effects are generally opposite to those of hyperthyroidism. It can lead to fatigue, irregular weight gain, puffiness in the limbs and face, and a slowed heart rate. It may also induce mood irregularities, such as depression. Because of the lowered thyroid activity, you may frequently feel colder than those around you. Both hypothyroidism and hyperthyroidism require you to make diet and lifestyle changes in order to prevent them from developing or lessen symptoms once they develop.

Chapter 2: How to Avoid Inflammation

Inflammation can have a severe impact on your ability to live your life as you desire by introducing painful symptoms and dangerous health conditions. Related pain can range from nearly negligible to debilitating, but all pain is symptomatic of more serious conditions inside the body, and allowing chronic inflammation to persist without exploring treatment options can worsen this pain. Inflammation should not be allowed to continue untreated when it occurs, as it may develop into more serious health problems. Make the change to an anti-inflammatory lifestyle as early as possible to combat these developments.

In order to take steps to fight back against pain, remember that inflammation is treatable, and you have the opportunity to greatly reduce how often it occurs or entirely rid yourself of it. This can often be accomplished through small lifestyle changes, like exercise and other adjustments. One of the most important treatments for inflammation is changing your diet. By consuming fewer ingredients that promote inflammation in the body, you can restrict how often chronic inflammation is able to hold you back. Replace them with healthy, anti-inflammatory alternatives that have been shown to greatly reduce the frequency of inflammation. Incorporate foods high in antioxidants into your diet, which counteract harmful oxidizing agents in foods and protect against cell damage. By making these changes, you develop methods for managing inflammation when it occurs. Over time, you will experience a notable change in how often you have pain and swelling.

A Manageable Condition

Though chronic inflammation can be difficult to deal with, it is a manageable condition. You do not have to live with painful symptoms forever, and inflammation does not always result in more serious health conditions if addressed as early as possible. You can regain control over your symptoms, giving you back freedom and mobility in your life even through small changes. There are steps you can take to lessen the role inflammation plays in your life, and they begin with lifestyle changes, such as dietary alterations.

You get out of your body what you put into it. Eating a diet full of unhealthy ingredients, like sugars and saturated fats, will worsen the symptoms. On the other hand, making an effort to restrict these ingredients can diminish and, in some cases, completely eliminate health problems such as weight gain and metabolism-related disorders. This is also true when it comes to inflammation. Studies indicate that "there is a substantial amount of evidence to suggest that many foods, nutrients and non-nutrient food components modulate inflammation both acutely and chronically," so changing what you eat can directly affect the frequency of harmful inflammation (Minihane et al., 2015, para. 17). While this does mean that the best way to tackle inflammation is to cut certain ingredients out of your diet, which can be tough initially, it also means that you can prevent chronic inflammation flare-ups and treatment by just adjusting your meals.

Certain foods can worsen inflammation, while others help to prevent it. It is best to avoid ingredients like sugars, refined carbs, and highly processed foods on an anti-inflammatory diet. These ingredients promote the development of harmful free radicals in the body, which have been linked to aging and diseases. Additionally, research has uncovered that "free radicals [...] are playing a relevant role in the pathogenesis of inflammation" and should be reduced as much as possible (Tomasi, Özben, and Skulachev, 2003, pg. v). However, foods with high antioxidant content help to counteract these free radicals and should be added to your diet to fight inflammation.

What Foods to Avoid

Sugar has become abundant in the food we eat every day, but consuming high amounts of sugar can be very dangerous, especially if you suffer from chronic inflammation. Excess sugar can even develop into insulin resistance and health complications like diabetes. Sugar and other chemical sweeteners (e.g., fructose) are the leading causes of inflammation, and these compounds are present in nearly every prepackaged food. Avoiding sugar usually means making a commitment to reading labels before you buy products, as well as cooking with whole ingredients. Natural sources of sugar, such as fruits, honey, and maple syrup, are much easier for your body to digest and do not generally result in inflammation. It is primarily refined sugars that should be cut out of your diet. This also includes sugary drinks, such as soda, some energy drinks, and juices with added sugar.

Saturated fats and oils can also increase the frequency of inflammation flare-ups. They tend to trigger inflammation of the fat tissue, which can worsen pain and lead to the development of heart conditions. While not all fats are bad for you, those linked to inflammation should not be consumed frequently if at all. Cut down on dairy products, especially cheese, as they are high in saturated fat. Also, limit your intake of omega-6 fatty acids, which are present in soy and vegetable oils. Avoid trans fats, which are common to fried foods, shelf-stable baked goods, and many snack foods.

Refined grains and carbs can also be dangerous when it comes to inflammation. Processed foods are typically full of these kinds of carbs, which can also lead to weight gain if consumed in excess. Refined carbs are those that have been processed after being harvested and do not appear naturally. It is always better to eat whole foods rather than processed grains. These kinds of carbs are typically high in gluten and have a high glycemic index, making them dangerous for people with diabetes and increasing the risk of inflammation in your gut and conditions like IBD. While you want to include some carbs in your diet, avoid anything made with white flour or white rice, and stick to whole grains and high-fiber carbs.

Processed meats are another source of inflammation. This includes bacon, ham, sausage, and hot dogs. It also includes smoked meats and processed meat snacks, such as jerky and smoked sausages. The inflammation resulting from eating high volumes of processed meat has been linked most frequently to colon cancer, so these meats should be eliminated in an anti-inflammatory diet. While not as great of a concern as processed meats, your consumption of red meat should also be reduced, though the occasional meal made with a lean cut of beef is all right. Select leaner proteins and white meat instead when possible.

Processed snack foods are also undesirable on the anti-inflammatory diet. Aside from inflammation, these foods are often loaded with unhealthy ingredients and preservatives to keep them shelf-stable. They are full of previously discussed ingredients to be avoided, like refined carbs and processed meats. They are frequently high in bad fats and sugars and can lead to weight gain if not replaced with healthy, fresh snack options.

While it may not seem immediately apparent, excessive drinking can also contribute to inflammation. Alcohol has been shown to raise inflammation markers in the body and cause injury in the liver and gut, which can lead to more serious health complications. Frequent alcohol consumption can impact how your organs interact with each other, reducing efficiency and often resulting in long-lasting organ damage. It can also cause inflammation in the brain, resulting in neurological conditions. Additionally, mixed drinks often involve liquids that have been sweetened with hidden sugars. Any alcohol consumption should be restricted to moderate amounts at most to avoid inflammation and related health conditions.

What Foods Can Help

It may sound like the anti-inflammatory diet has just restricted all foods, but don't despair; there are plenty of healthy and delicious ingredients that help to fight off inflammation in the body. These foods are often high in antioxidants or have otherwise been shown to reduce inflammation and related symptoms.

Anti-inflammatory diets should be high in leafy greens. This includes kale, spinach, cabbage, collard greens, chard, and arugula. These vegetables have high vitamin and mineral concentration, especially vitamins A, C, and K. They are packed with antioxidants and can be extremely versatile in recipes. They can be incorporated into almost any dish as a base or side. Even just a cup of sautéed spinach with dinner can help to prevent heart disease and lower cholesterol. Leafy greens also contain a compound called quercetin, which is a natural anti-inflammatory that can help reduce pain.

Nuts are high in healthy fats and very low in saturated and trans fats. They help to fight against inflammation, and many are high in vitamin E, which can help rid the body of free radicals. Almonds, walnuts, pecans, hazelnuts, pistachios, cashews, Brazil nuts, and macadamia nuts are all excellent options to add to your diet. They can be incorporated as a topping on all sorts of meals or even eaten by the handful as a quick and healthy snack on a busy day.

Tomatoes are also a great option for fighting against inflammation. They are high in vitamins and minerals like potassium, vitamin C, and antioxidants. They also contain high amounts of fiber to support healthy digestion, and they have been linked to reducing the risk of cardiovascular diseases. Note that there have been some claims that nightshade vegetables (e.g., tomatoes, potatoes, and eggplant) can increase inflammation, but these claims are generally not supported by research. Tomatoes are full of benefits for anti-inflammatory diets and should be included in most circumstances. However, pay attention to your own body and limit nightshades if necessary.

While saturated fats and trans fats should be avoided, healthy fats are great for anti-inflammation and making meals filling. Neglecting fats altogether can lead to diets higher in sugars and carbs, which can lead to inflammation. Instead, eat a good amount of healthy fats, like omega-3s. These fats are commonly found in seafood, nuts, avocados, eggs, and even dark chocolate. Fish like salmon and sardines are especially high in healthy omega-3 fatty acids. They also come from cooking oils like olive oil and avocado oil. Olive oil is frequently used in meal plans like the Mediterranean diet and keto diet because of its healthy properties when it comes to blood pressure and heart disease, but it is also full of antioxidants like vitamins E and K.

Many types of berries are also high in antioxidants. You should include a serving of fresh berries in your diet frequently in your daily meals, even on their own as a snack. You can use blueberries, raspberries, blackberries, strawberries, cranberries, acai berries, or any other berry. It is best to incorporate a variety of berries into your diet to get the best benefits. Cherries, while not technically berries, also have similar anti-inflammatory power. While berries also contain sugar, the sugar from whole foods is not as great of a concern as refined and added sugars as it can be metabolized easier, and their health benefits greatly outweigh their sugar content. In fact, they can be used as a way to naturally sweeten foods like yogurt, breakfast bowls, and smoothies.

Green vegetables are generally healthy options, and broccoli is no outlier. Broccoli contains an antioxidant known as sulforaphane, which is adept at preventing inflammation. It also contains vitamins C and K, as well as high amounts of calcium, which is important in a diet that restricts high-fat dairy.

Broccoli pairs well with garlic and ginger, which are also anti-inflammatory ingredients.

Avocados have recently become known as a bit of a superfood. This is because they have such a wide variety of health benefits. They are full of healthy monounsaturated fatty acids, as well as plenty of vitamins and minerals for a healthy diet. They are high in nutrients, and just a little bit of avocado goes a long way. Avocados support healthy heart functions, contain folate that the body uses to prevent the development of cancers, and improve digestion. Their benefits in an anti-inflammatory diet are immense, and you'll want to add them whenever you can. Luckily, this is made easy by their creamy texture and great taste.

If you drink soda for the caffeinated energy boost, consider ditching it in favor of green tea. Green tea is high in caffeine but low in sugar, which means you can get energy without the dangers of a high sugar diet or the concerns of a sugar crash. It is full of inflammation-fighting antioxidants and has been linked to faster rates of burning fat during exercise. If green tea isn't to your taste, you can also drink no-sugar-added fruit juices (e.g., pineapple and cherry juice) or add anti-inflammatory spices to tea (e.g., ginger, cinnamon, and turmeric).

Tips for Busy Lifestyles

You may be tempted to believe that eating healthy is only for people with a great deal of free time and that you simply do not have the time to cook healthy meals each day. However, there are plenty of ways to cut down on inflammatory foods that do not require a large time commitment. There are many antioxidant-rich recipes that can be prepared in as little as 10 minutes, and on the days when time is especially tight, meals prepared in advance can help to ensure you always find time to eat right. If you have a busy lifestyle, follow these tips to correct your eating habits without any extra time spent.

Meal Prep

If you are routinely busy on weekdays but you have more free time on weekends or regularly scheduled days off, consider meal prepping at the beginning of each week. This involves preparing food ahead of time so that, on a busy day, you can simply heat and eat. Complete recipes all the way up to the cooking stage on the weekends, or make dinners large enough to have leftovers for the rest of the week. Then if you return home from work too exhausted to cook, you have a healthy meal waiting for you that takes less time and effort than a TV dinner. Meal prepping works best if you cook a variety of meals over the weekend so that you do not end up eating leftovers of the same dish every day.

Don't Skip Meals

If you're running late as you leave the house early in the morning, it may be tempting to simply skip a meal, but this is not a good idea. The old adage of breakfast being the most important meal of the day is actually true. Breakfast can help you kick start your metabolism in the morning, aiding in weight loss and healthy digestion. Breakfast is also a good way to help your body wake up for the day, and eating a balanced and healthy meal can help you get into the right headspace to tackle the day's events. Additionally, making breakfast does not have to take up much time, even while avoiding inflammatory foods. While you don't want to eat toast or sugary cereal, there are plenty of quick and easy breakfast recipes in this book that only take 5–10 minutes and can be taken with you on your daily commute.

Time-Saving Recipes

Recipes that save you time are your best friends. Many of the recipes below are written with a busy schedule in mind and cut out unnecessary and slow steps in favor of faster alternatives. While your health is valuable, your time is too, and the key to changing your diet on a time crunch is respecting both aspects and selecting meals that work best for the amount of time you are able to spend on them. Additionally, switching to a less inflammatory diet can actually save you time in the long run as pain and swelling from inflammation decreases. You will be able to waste less time in pain and spend more time doing what you love.

Chapter 3: Breakfast

Breakfast can set the tone for the rest of the day. Use these recipes to start your mornings right and get off on the right foot, no matter what the rest of the day entails. Smoothies are perfect for grab-and-go breakfasts, while omelets and ancient grains make hearty, filling meals minus all the refined carbs.

Smoothies

Strawberry Almond Milk Smoothie

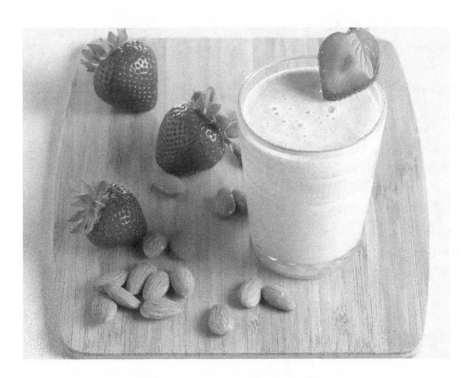

When in a rush, smoothies can be a perfect option for a quick breakfast. This smoothie takes just 5 minutes to prepare, leaving you with more time to get ready to start the day in the morning without skipping out on a healthy breakfast. A strawberry almond milk smoothie packs plenty of protein and energy that will last you until lunchtime. Strawberries and almonds are both great anti-inflammatory ingredients that taste amazing in a nice refreshing smoothie. Together with a little bit of honey, you won't even notice the lack of added sugar.

Nutritional Information:

- Calories: 130
- Total fat: 6 g
- Total carbohydrates: 15 g
- Sugar: 9 g
- Fiber: 3 g
- Protein: 6 g
- Sodium: 130 mg

Time: 5 minutes

Serving Size: 8 ounces (yields 2 servings)

Ingredients:

- ¾ cup almond milk, unsweetened
- 1 cup strawberries, frozen or chilled
- ¼ cup plain yogurt, unsweetened
- 1 tablespoon honey
- 1 tablespoon almond butter

Directions:

1. Add almond milk, strawberries, and yogurt to blender.
2. Blend for 30 seconds to combine ingredients.
3. Add honey and almond butter.
4. Blend in 30-second intervals until smoothie reaches desired consistency.

Pitaya Smoothie

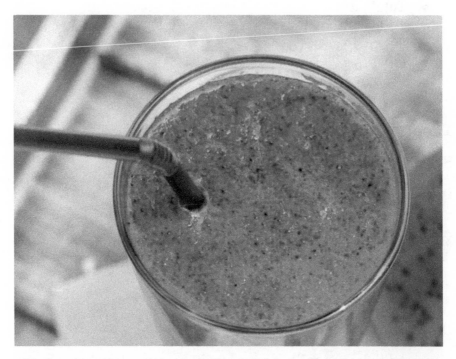

Pitaya, also known as dragon fruit, is a great base for anti-inflammatory recipes. It is high in antioxidants, which help to reduce inflammation and prevent cell damage. It is also low in calories while still being high in vitamins, minerals, and fiber, making it a great healthy option for a smoothie.

If you've never worked with pitaya before, don't be intimidated by its odd looks. It is commonly available in most grocery stores frozen and cubed, so you don't have to worry about how to prepare fresh pitaya. This smoothie takes full advantage of the frozen fruit and cuts out the need to blend ice, which can be difficult for some blenders. This recipe is especially easy and convenient, only requiring you to measure and blend for a great-tasting smoothie you can take for an on-the-go breakfast.

Nutritional Information:

- Calories: 132
- Total fat: 1.1 g
- Total carbohydrates: 30 g
- Sugar: 17 g
- Fiber: 5 g
- Protein: 3 g
- Sodium: 48 mg

Time: 5 minutes

Serving Size: 8 ounces (yields 1 serving)

Ingredients:

- ¼ cup almond milk, unsweetened
- ¼ cup dragon fruit, frozen and cubed or chunked
- ¼ cup mango, frozen and cubed or chunked
- ¼ cup strawberries, frozen
- ½ banana, sliced

Directions:

1. Add almond milk, dragon fruit, mango, strawberries, and banana to blender.
2. Blend in 30-second increments until desired consistency is reached.

Eggs

Spinach and Tomato Omelet

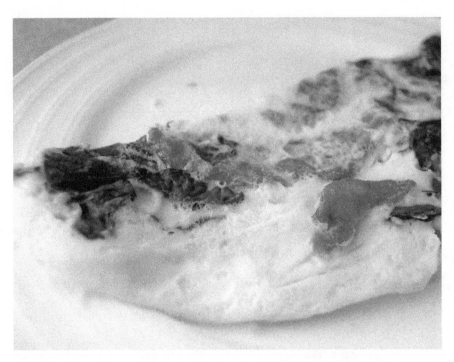

Eggs are a great way to step away from grains and gluten for breakfast. They provide a filling meal without ingredients that can cause or worsen inflammation. Making an omelet is easy and fast, but if you find your omelet losing its shape, this recipe can also be turned into scrambled eggs in a pinch. Cherry tomatoes are convenient to have around for snacking and are much easier to chop up than their larger counterparts, but either type can be used.

Nutritional Information:

- Calories: 207
- Total fat: 50 g
- Total carbohydrates: 6 g
- Sugar: 2 g
- Fiber: 2 g
- Protein: 16 g
- Sodium: 667 mg

Time: 15 minutes

Serving Size: 1 omelet (yields 1 serving)

Ingredients:

- 2 eggs
- ¼ cup water
- 1 cup baby spinach
- ¼ cup cherry tomatoes
- 3 tablespoons olive oil
- ¼ teaspoon salt
- ¼ teaspoon ground black pepper

Directions:

1. Wash cherry tomatoes and cut into halves or slices. Chop baby spinach.
2. Add 1 tablespoon oil to the pan. On medium heat, fry the tomatoes until tender, around 2 minutes. Remove tomatoes from the pan and set aside.
3. Crack eggs into a small bowl and add salt, pepper, and water. Beat with a fork until combined, and stir in baby spinach.
4. Add 2 tablespoons of oil to the pan over medium heat and pour in the egg mixture. Tilt the pan so that the eggs settle evenly.
5. With a spatula, gently push the edges of the cooked eggs away from the sides of the pan, unsticking them and allowing any uncooked egg to reach the pan's surface.

Continue cooking for 2–3 minutes until there is nearly no runny egg left.

6. Once the omelet has mostly solidified, add fried tomatoes to one side and fold the opposite end of the omelet over using a spatula. Press gently to stick the ends together. Remove the omelet from the pan and serve.

Gluten-Free Grains

Turmeric Cinnamon Oatmeal

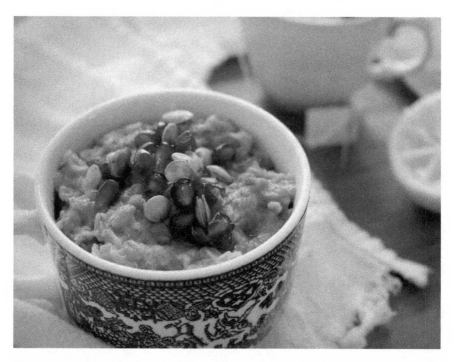

Oats are a great gluten-free grain option for breakfast. By using quick-cook oats, you can cut down on cook time dramatically and make a filling breakfast that's ready in minutes. The added turmeric, cinnamon, and ginger add to this recipe's anti-inflammatory properties.

Nutritional Information:

- Calories: 471
- Total fat: 32 g
- Total carbohydrates: 43 g
- Sugar: 5 g
- Fiber: 10 g
- Protein: 12 g
- Sodium: 24 mg

Time: 5 minutes

Serving Size: 1 cup (yields 2 servings)

Ingredients:

- 1 cup quick cook oats
- 1⅓ cups coconut milk
- ½ teaspoon ginger, ground or grated
- 1 teaspoon cinnamon
- 1 teaspoon ground turmeric

Directions:

1. Take a microwave-safe bowl and add oats and coconut milk.
2. Microwave on high for 1 minute.
3. Add in ginger, cinnamon, and turmeric. Stir to combine.
4. Microwave for another minute, stirring in 30-second intervals.

Sweet Maple Rice Porridge

If you're craving something sweet and hearty without risking inflammation, try this sweet maple rice porridge. Maple syrup is high in antioxidants and makes for a tasty anti-inflammatory sweetener. When baked in the oven, it gets the blackberries and peaches perfectly caramelized.

Nutritional Information:

- Calories: 324
- Total fat: 2 g
- Total carbohydrates: 73 g
- Sugar: 28 g
- Fiber: 6 g
- Protein: 5 g
- Sodium: 15 mg

Time: 30 minutes

Serving Size: 1 cup (yields 1 serving)

Ingredients:

- ½ cup brown rice
- 1 cup water
- ¼ cup blackberries
- ½ peach, sliced
- 2 tablespoons pure maple syrup
- ½ teaspoon cinnamon
- ¼ teaspoon nutmeg

Directions:

1. Preheat oven to 400 degrees Fahrenheit.
2. Add rice and water to a pot. Bring to a boil over medium-high heat, around 2 minutes.
3. Add cinnamon and nutmeg, and stir to incorporate.

4. Cover the pot and lower heat to medium. Simmer for 10–12 minutes until tender.
5. Transfer cooked rice to an oven-safe bowl. Add blackberries and peaches, and drizzle maple syrup on top.
6. Bake it in the oven for 10–15 minutes until it bubbles and the fruit is caramelized.

Ancient Grains Breakfast Bowl

Grains high in gluten, such as wheat and rye, can worsen inflammation, taking cereal and toast off the breakfast table. Replace them with gluten-free grains, such as millet and buckwheat, with this ancient grains breakfast bowl. This recipe uses strawberries and blueberries, but you can add or substitute inflammation-fighting fruits of your choice, such as apples, cherries, or blackberries.

Nutritional Information:

- Calories: 211
- Total fat: 3 g
- Total carbohydrates: 39 g
- Sugar: 1 g
- Fiber: 3 g
- Protein: 4 g
- Sodium: 107 mg

Time: 30 minutes

Serving Size: 1 cup (yields 4 servings)

Ingredients:

- ½ cup millet
- ½ cup buckwheat
- 2½ cups almond milk, unsweetened
- ¼ cup strawberries, sliced
- ¼ cup blueberries
- ½ teaspoon ground cinnamon

- ¼ teaspoon ground clove

Directions:

1. Add millet, buckwheat, and almond milk to a saucepan.
2. Bring to a boil on high heat. Once boiling, reduce heat to medium-low and cover.
3. Cook until grains are tender, around 20–25 minutes.
4. Remove from heat and transfer to a bowl. Add cinnamon and clove, and mix to combine.
5. Place strawberries and blueberries on top, sprinkle with more cinnamon, and serve.

Chapter 4: Salads and Side Dishes

Whether you are looking to complement a meal or simply enjoy one of these dishes as a quick lunch, these salads and side dishes are nutritional powerhouses and pack plenty of flavors too. "Healthy" doesn't have to mean devoid of flavor. These salads are tasty on their own or paired with a homemade dressing. Either way, you won't feel like you're on a diet while eating them, and the sides are so good they can stand on their own.

Salads

Kale and Berry Salad

Eating a healthy salad doesn't have to be a chore with this kale and berry salad recipe. Kale provides this salad with high levels of anti-inflammatory omega-3s. Berries keep the overall flavor sweet without needing to add dressing, but the salad also pairs well with a turmeric dressing if preferred.

Nutritional Information:

- Calories: 141
- Total fat: 8 g
- Total carbohydrates: 17 g
- Sugar: 7 g
- Fiber: 6 g
- Protein: 6 g
- Sodium: 15 mg

Time: 10 minutes

Serving Size: 1 cup (yields 2 servings)

Ingredients:

- 2 cups kale
- ½ cup carrots, shredded
- ½ cup blueberries
- ¼ cup cherries
- ¼ cup almonds, sliced
- 1 tablespoon pumpkin seeds
- 1 tablespoon toasted sesame seeds

Directions:

1. Rinse and chop kale, taking care to remove and discard the tough stems.
2. Move kale to a large bowl. Halve cherries, removing the pits.
3. Add shredded carrots, blueberries, halved cherries, and almonds to the large bowl and toss until evenly distributed. Mix in almonds, pumpkin seeds, and sesame seeds.

Avocado Salad

Avocados are often cited as a superfood for their wide variety of health benefits. They boast plenty of healthy fats and antioxidants and can help your body greatly diminish inflammation. Combined with their rich flavor and creamy texture, this avocado salad is both nutritious and delicious.

Nutritional Information:

- Calories: 292
- Total fat: 33 g
- Total carbohydrates: 17 g
- Sugar: 5 g
- Fiber: 10 g
- Protein: 11 g

- Sodium: 172 mg

Time: 10 minutes

Serving Size: 1 cup (yields 2 servings)

Ingredients:

- 1½ cups spinach
- 1 avocado
- 1 orange
- 2 ounces goat cheese
- ¼ cup walnuts, chopped

Directions:

1. Wash and chop spinach and transfer it to a large bowl.
2. Cut the avocado in half lengthwise, rotating as you cut to avoid the pit, and twist to separate into halves. Remove the pit with a large spoon. Then use the spoon to scoop out the remaining avocado halves and slice.
3. Peel the orange, then pull apart into sections, or use a knife to slice if thinner pieces are desired.
4. Add avocado and orange slices to spinach, shaking to mix. Top with crumbled goat cheese and chopped walnuts.

Quinoa and Black Bean Salad

Eating a salad doesn't have to mean limiting yourself to just fruits and veggies. This quinoa and black bean salad incorporates gluten-free ancient grains and plenty of protein from the beans to make a hearty, filling meal.

Nutritional Information:

- Calories: 231
- Total fat: 2 g
- Total carbohydrates: 41 g
- Sugar: 4 g
- Fiber: 13 g

- Protein: 13 g
- Sodium: 779 mg

Time: 25 minutes

Serving Size: 1 cup (yields 3 servings)

Ingredients:

- 2 cups kale
- 1 can (15 ounces) black beans
- ½ cup carrots, shredded
- 1 cup quinoa
- 2 cups vegetable broth
- 1 tablespoon garlic, minced
- ½ lemon

Directions:

1. Rinse and drain quinoa, then transfer it to a pot on the stove. Add vegetable broth and garlic, and stir.
2. Bring to a boil over medium-high heat, around 2 minutes. Reduce heat to low and cover. Simmer for 18–20 minutes or until all liquid has been absorbed into the quinoa.
3. Rinse and chop kale, discarding the tough stems, and transfer it to a large bowl.
4. Open the can of black beans. Rinse and drain twice.
5. Mix in quinoa, carrots, and black beans. Top with a squeeze of lemon juice.

Sides

Caramelized Butternut Squash

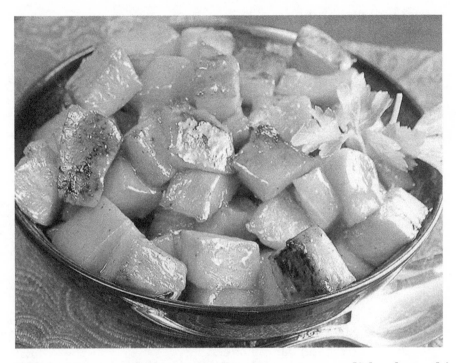

Butternut squash is typically an autumn dish, but this caramelized butternut squash recipe is so good you'll find yourself serving it in all seasons. Squash is also a bountiful source of vitamin E, vitamin C, and beta carotene, which are all antioxidants.

Nutritional Information:

- Calories: 44
- Total fat: 4 g
- Total carbohydrates: 4 g
- Sugar: 2 g
- Fiber: <1 g
- Protein: <1 g
- Sodium: 292 mg

Time: 40 minutes

Serving Size: ½ cup (yields 8 servings)

Ingredients:

- 1 butternut squash
- 1 tablespoon pure maple syrup
- 2 tablespoons olive oil
- ½ teaspoon ground turmeric
- 1 teaspoon salt
- 1 teaspoon paprika

Directions:

1. Preheat oven to 375 degrees Fahrenheit.
2. Using a large knife, slice off the top and bottom ends of the butternut squash. With a vegetable peeler, peel until the darker orange flesh is visible.
3. Stand the squash up vertically on the cutting board, and slice in half. Use a spoon to remove seeds. Cut the squash into slices, and then dice to form cubes.
4. In a bowl, toss squash with olive oil, turmeric, salt, and paprika until well coated.
5. Cover a baking sheet with aluminum foil. Spread coated squash over the baking sheet.
6. Roast in the oven for 20 minutes, stirring in 10-minute intervals.
7. Remove squash from the oven. Drizzle with maple syrup, then return to oven and cook for another 12–15 minutes until maple syrup caramelizes.

Roasted Radishes

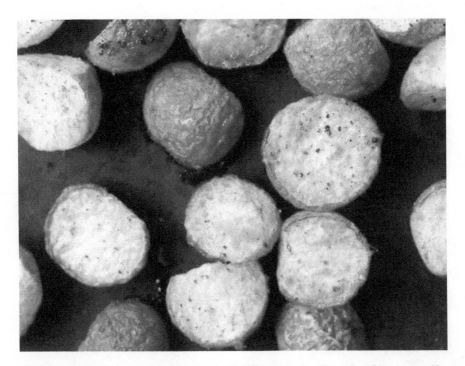

Radishes are a good source of fiber and vitamin C, as well as anti-inflammatory agents. Raw radishes are most common to salads, but when roasted, their flavor changes entirely, and they become similar to potatoes.

Nutritional Information:

- Calories: 82
- Total fat: 5 g
- Total carbohydrates: 8 g
- Sugar: 4 g
- Fiber: 4 g
- Protein: <1 g
- Sodium: 47 1 mg

Time: 40 minutes

Serving Size: ½ cup (yields 3 servings)

Ingredients:

- 1½ cups radishes, around 3 bunches
- 1 tablespoon olive oil
- ¼ lemon
- 1 teaspoon garlic powder
- 1 teaspoon dried rosemary
- ½ teaspoon salt
- ½ teaspoon ground black pepper

Directions:

1. Preheat oven to 350 degrees Fahrenheit.
2. Wash radishes and transfer to cutting board. Cut off stems and roots. Cut into quarters.
3. Move radishes to a medium-size bowl and add oil, salt, and pepper.
4. Line a baking sheet with aluminum foil. Spread radishes over the baking sheet.
5. Cook in the oven for 15 minutes. Remove from the oven, stir, and cook for another 15 minutes.
6. Sprinkle with garlic powder, dried rosemary, and lemon juice. Return to oven for 5 minutes or until tender.

Zucchini Rice

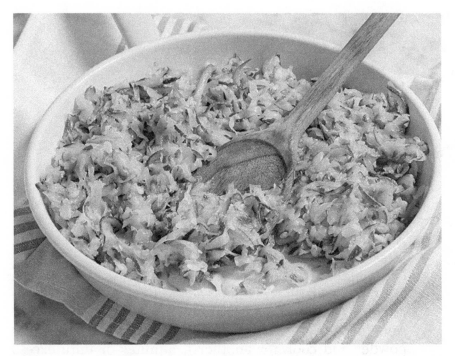

White rice is a highly processed food that can cause inflammation and should be avoided on an anti-inflammatory diet. If you find yourself missing it, however, try this zucchini rice instead for a healthy and anti-inflammatory alternative.

Nutritional Information:

- Calories: 52
- Total fat: 4 g
- Total carbohydrates: 6 g
- Sugar: 5 g
- Fiber: 2 g
- Protein: 2 g
- Sodium: 10 mg

Time: 15 minutes

Serving Size: ½ cup (yields 4 servings)

Ingredients:

- 2 large zucchini
- ½ white onion
- 1 tablespoon olive oil
- ½ teaspoon salt
- ½ teaspoon garlic powder

Directions:

1. Cut off the top and bottom ends of the zucchini. Using a spiralizer, spiralize zucchini. Alternatively, you can slice the zucchini into thin slices by hand.
2. Add zucchini to a food processor and pulse in 20-second intervals until zucchini pieces are rice-sized.
3. Dice onion into fine pieces.
4. Heat olive oil in a skillet and add onions. Sauté over medium heat until tender, around 5 minutes.
5. Add zucchini to the skillet. Sprinkle with salt and garlic powder and cook for another 5 minutes or until excess moisture has been cooked off.

Sweet potatoes are a great addition to any anti-inflammatory repertoire. They are high in antioxidants, namely vitamin C, vitamin E, and alpha and beta carotene. They are also packed with flavor, which you can take full advantage of with this sweet potato quinoa recipe.

Nutritional Information:

- Calories: 188
- Total fat: 8 g
- Total carbohydrates: 26 g
- Sugar: 4 g
- Fiber: 4 g
- Protein: 4 g
- Sodium: 668 mg

Time: 25 minutes

Serving Size: 1 cup (yields 4 servings)

Ingredients:

- 2 sweet potatoes
- 1 cup quinoa
- 2 cups kale
- 2 cups vegetable broth
- 2 tablespoons olive oil
- 1 tablespoon garlic, minced
- 1 tablespoon apple cider vinegar
- 2 tablespoons fresh chervil
- ¼ teaspoon salt
- ¼ teaspoon ground black pepper

Directions:

1. Cut ends off sweet potatoes, peel, and dice into ¼-inch chunks.
2. Add olive oil and sweet potatoes to a skillet. Sauté over medium-high heat for 2 minutes.
3. Add in quinoa and garlic, as well as apple cider vinegar, salt, and pepper. Cook for another 2 minutes.
4. Turn heat to low and add vegetable broth. Stir to combine, then cover and allow to cook for 12 minutes.
5. Uncover and stir in kale and chervil. Cook for 3 minutes, ensuring all ingredients are tender and well-combined, and then serve.

Chapter 5: Dressings and Other Condiments

Most dressings and condiments you can buy from the store are loaded with added sugars. In order to avoid these, it's best to use your own homemade toppings. Luckily, even if you have never tried to make your own dressing before, these recipes are easy to prepare and require little time to make. Use them to produce great flavors for dressing up your favorite salads, proteins, and sides.

Dressings

Turmeric Dressing

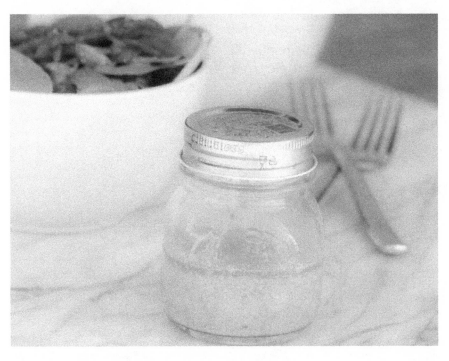

Turmeric dressing pairs well with just about any salad to give it a boost in antioxidants. It is packed with healthy fats and great flavor, so you can feel like you're indulging without sacrificing any health benefits.

Nutritional Information:

- Calories: 662
- Total fat: 72 g
- Total carbohydrates: 6 g
- Sugar: 1 g
- Fiber: 2 g
- Protein: 1 g
- Sodium: 782 mg

Time: 5 minutes

Serving Size: ¾ cup (yields 1 serving)

Ingredients:

- ⅓ cup olive oil
- 1 teaspoon turmeric
- ½ teaspoon garlic powder
- 2 tablespoons apple cider vinegar
- 1 teaspoon ginger, ground or grated
- ½ lemon
- 1 teaspoon parsley
- ½ teaspoon pink Himalayan salt
- ½ teaspoon ground black pepper

Directions:

1. In a blender, add olive oil, turmeric, garlic powder, apple cider vinegar, and ginger.
2. Squeeze in the juice from the lemon. Ensure all seeds are removed.
3. Finely chop the parsley, and add to blender.
4. Grind in pink Himalayan salt and black pepper.
5. Blend for 30 seconds until smooth and creamy.

Balsamic Vinaigrette

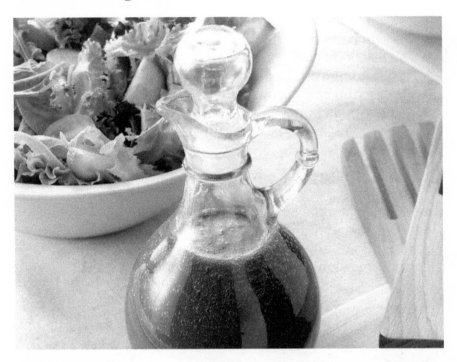

Balsamic vinaigrette is a stand-out tangy option for lots of flavor with only a little work. Balsamic vinegar fights inflammation, and it is notably antiviral and antibacterial. When added to an anti-inflammatory salad, this recipe provides a powerful antioxidant boost.

Nutritional Information:

- Calories: 1,034
- Total fat: 108 g
- Total carbohydrates: 16 g
- Sugar: 14 g
- Fiber: 1 g
- Protein: 1 g
- Sodium: 75 mg

Time: 5 minutes

Serving Size: ½ cup (yields 1 serving)

Ingredients:

- ½ cup olive oil
- ¼ cup balsamic vinegar
- ½ teaspoon garlic powder
- 1 teaspoon fresh basil
- 1 teaspoon spicy brown mustard
- ½ teaspoon honey

Directions:

1. To a blender, add olive oil, balsamic vinegar, and garlic powder.
2. Finely chop the basil and add to the mix.
3. Pour in honey and spicy brown mustard.
4. Blend in 10-second intervals for 30 seconds. The dressing should look well-combined.

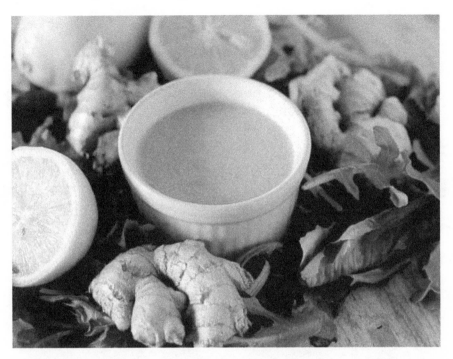

This lemon-ginger dressing is great for detoxification. With plenty of bold flavor and zest, you'll be tempted to use it not just for salads — you can also use it as a veggie dip, or you can even drizzle it over a lean protein.

Nutritional Information:

- Calories: 430
- Total fat: 43 g
- Total carbohydrates: 19 g
- Sugar: 4 g
- Fiber: 4 g
- Protein: 2 g
- Sodium: 19 mg

Time: 5 minutes

Serving Size: ½ cup (yields 1 serving)

Ingredients:

- 2 lemons
- 3 tablespoons olive oil
- 1 teaspoon garlic powder
- 2 teaspoon ground turmeric
- 2 teaspoon ginger, ground or grated
- ¼ teaspoon ground black pepper

Directions:

1. Cut lemons in half. Juice into a blender, making sure all seeds are removed.
2. Add in olive oil, garlic powder, turmeric, ginger, and black pepper.
3. Blend for 20 seconds, just until combined.

Condiments

Barbecue Sauce

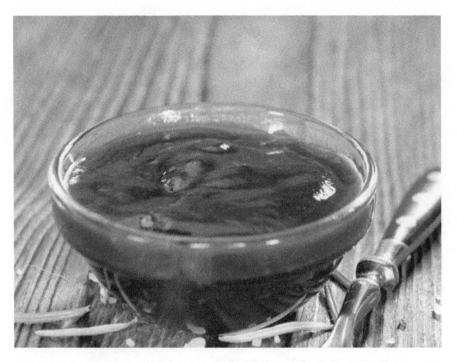

Normal barbecue sauce may be filled with inflammatory sugar, but it doesn't mean you have to give up barbecue altogether. Instead, replace it with this recipe for a delicious, healthy alternative.

Nutritional Information:

- Calories: 42
- Total fat: <1 g
- Total carbohydrates: 9 g
- Sugar: 6 g
- Fiber: 2 g
- Protein: 2 g
- Sodium: 274 mg

Time: 25 minutes

Serving Size: ½ cup (yields 4 servings)

Ingredients:

- 1½ cups vegetable stock
- 1 white onion
- 1 can (6 ounces) tomato paste
- 2 tablespoons apple cider vinegar
- 2 tablespoons garlic, minced
- 1 teaspoon honey
- 1 tablespoon olive oil
- 1 tablespoon soy sauce
- 1 teaspoon mustard
- 1 teaspoon ground red pepper
- 1 teaspoon basil, chopped

Directions:

1. Dice onion into fine pieces.
2. To a saucepan on the stove, add olive oil and diced onion. Sauté over medium-high heat until soft, around 3–4 minutes.
3. Pour in vegetable stock, tomato paste, and apple cider vinegar. Stir to combine. Add garlic, honey, soy sauce, mustard, ground red pepper, and basil. Heat for 1 minute to thin honey, and then stir.
4. Bring sauce to a boil on medium heat, around 4 minutes.
5. Decrease the heat to low and cover. Let the sauce simmer for 20 minutes to thicken, stirring every 5 minutes to ensure no burning occurs.

Salsa Verde

Shelf-stable salsa can be full of inflammatory ingredients and unnatural preservatives. The next time you crave tacos, try this recipe for an anti-inflammatory homemade salsa verde that is even better than prepackaged salsas. You can use it to add flavor to tacos and chicken fajitas, or you can even eat it as a spicy topping or dip.

Nutritional Information:

- Calories: 28
- Total fat: 3 g
- Total carbohydrates: 2 g
- Sugar: 1 g
- Fiber: <1 g
- Protein: <1 g
- Sodium: 775 mg

Time: 30 minutes

Serving Size: ½ cup (yields 6 servings)

Ingredients:

- 1½ pounds tomatillos
- ½ yellow onion
- 1 jalapeno pepper
- 3 ounces cilantro, about 1 bunch
- 1 tablespoon olive oil
- 1 tablespoon garlic, minced
- 2 teaspoon salt

Directions:

1. Preheat oven to 375 degrees Fahrenheit.
2. Peel and wash tomatillos.
3. Line a baking sheet with tin foil. Spread tomatillos onto the sheet, saving space for the other ingredients.
4. Wash the jalapeno pepper and add it to the baking sheet.

5. Cut onion into thirds. With your hands, gently separate the layers onto the baking sheet. You do not have to fully separate all the layers, but each piece should be of a similar thickness.
6. Drizzle with olive oil and sprinkle with salt and garlic.
7. Roast all ingredients in the oven for 10–12 minutes. Tomatillos and jalapeno should be soft, and onion should be lightly browned.
8. Let cool for 10 minutes.
9. Transfer to a food processor or blender, and add cilantro. Blend until well mixed but slightly chunky, around 1 minute.

Chapter 6: Snacks

Processed and prepackaged snack foods (e.g., chips and cookies) are ill-suited to this diet, but these replacements are so good you won't miss them. Anti-inflammatory snacks come in a wide variety of forms. If you're looking for something with next-to-no prep time, try a simple handful of almonds or a cup of no-sugar-added applesauce. That said, the following recipes are all exceptionally quick to prepare as well and make for wonderful options to enjoy throughout the day.

Yogurt

Almond and Blueberry Yogurt

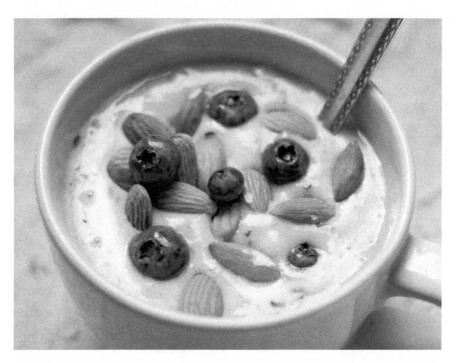

Simple and tasty, this almond and blueberry yogurt proves you don't have to spend a long time on healthy snacks. You can prepare this in just a few minutes and refrigerate in the morning, making for the perfect snack in the middle of a busy day. Yogurt is known to reduce inflammation, alongside the antioxidant-packed almonds and blueberries. This recipe uses regular nonfat yogurt, but you can swap it out for nonfat Greek yogurt if you prefer.

Nutritional Information:

- Calories: 197
- Total fat: 7 g
- Total carbohydrates: 23 g
- Sugar: 18 g
- Fiber: 4 g
- Protein: 13 g
- Sodium: 173 mg

Time: 2 minutes

Serving Size: ½ cup (yields 1 serving)

Ingredients:

- ¼ cup nonfat yogurt
- 1 tablespoon almonds, sliced
- ½ cup blueberries
- 1 teaspoon chia seeds

Directions:

1. Scoop yogurt into a bowl or to-go container.
2. Mix in almonds, blueberries, and chia seeds.

Strawberry Greek Yogurt

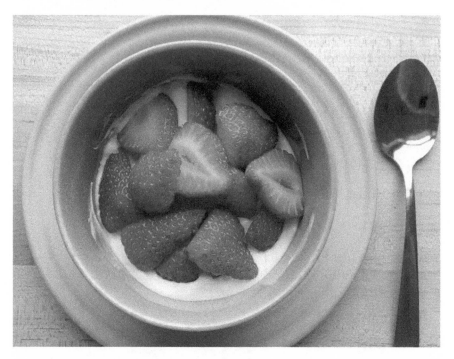

If you find yourself missing sweet treats, like ice cream sundaes, this strawberry Greek yogurt is sure to please. Made with just a touch of cacao powder, the yogurt stays sweet and chocolatey without needing to add in extra sugar.

Additionally, Greek yogurt boasts a variety of health benefits. It's a great source of calcium. It's chock-full of probiotics, and it's been linked to reducing the symptoms of conditions related to inflammation, such as high blood pressure and type 2 diabetes.

Nutritional Information:

- Calories: 170
- Total fat: 6 g
- Total carbohydrates: 20 g
- Sugar: 9 g
- Fiber: 5 g
- Protein: 10 g

- Sodium: 65 mg

Time: 5 minutes

Serving Size: ½ cup (yields 1 serving)

Ingredients:

- ¼ cup nonfat Greek yogurt
- 2 tablespoons cacao powder
- 1 tablespoon almonds, sliced
- ¼ cup strawberries, sliced
- ½ teaspoon cinnamon

Directions:

1. Scoop yogurt into a bowl or to-go container.
2. Add cacao powder and mix until powder is no longer visible.
3. Mix in almonds, strawberries, and cinnamon.

Smoothies

Matcha Smoothie

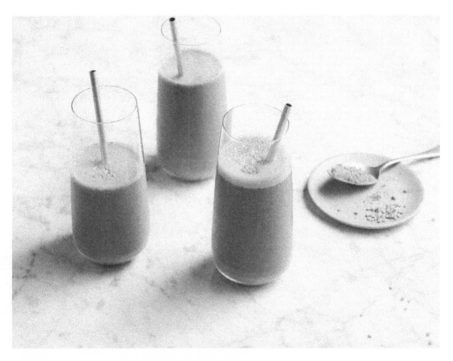

Matcha is a powdered version of green tea. It has all the health benefits of green tea, including its antioxidants and anti-inflammatory abilities, but in a convenient and versatile powdered form. Moreover, because it's powdered, all these benefits exist in much higher concentrations. For a great midday snack that makes use of this antioxidant powerhouse, try this matcha smoothie.

Nutritional Information:

- Calories: 402
- Total fat: 28 g
- Total carbohydrates: 43 g
- Sugar: 19 g

- Fiber: 9 g
- Protein: 8 g
- Sodium: 95 mg

Time: 5 minutes

Serving Size: 8 ounces (yields 1 serving)

Ingredients:

- ½ cup coconut milk
- 1 banana, sliced
- ½ cup spinach
- ¼ cup pineapple, chopped and frozen or chilled
- 1 teaspoon matcha powder
- ¼ cup raspberries, halved
- 1 teaspoon chia seeds

Directions:

1. Add coconut milk, banana, spinach, pineapple, and matcha powder to a blender.
2. Blend in 30-second increments until the desired thickness is reached.
3. Top with raspberries and chia seeds.

Light Snacks

Sweet Potato and Beet Hummus

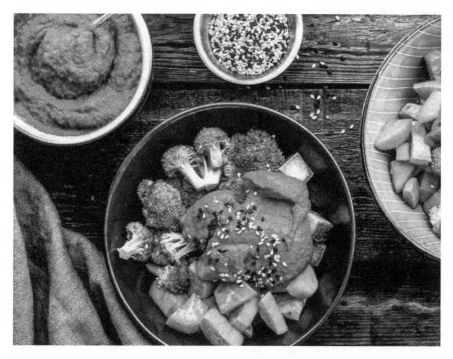

Hummus is full of healthy fats and plenty of protein from the chickpea base. The added sweet potatoes and beets used in this recipe gives the hummus a unique pink color without any added food coloring. Since this recipe takes a bit more prep time than some other snacks, it is best prepared over the weekend and enjoyed in portions throughout the week. Eat with carrot sticks, kale chips, or even on its own by the forkful.

Nutritional Information:

- Calories: 250
- Total fat: 17 g
- Total carbohydrates: 19 g
- Sugar: 5 g

- Fiber: 5 g
- Protein: 6 g
- Sodium: 948 mg

Time: 30 minutes

Serving Size: ½ cup (yields 4 servings)

Ingredients:

- ½ sweet potato
- 1 beet
- 1 can (15 ounces) chickpeas
- ¼ cup olive oil
- ¼ cup tahini
- 2 tablespoons garlic, minced
- 1 teaspoon turmeric
- 2 teaspoon pink Himalayan salt

Directions:

1. Wash, peel, and dice the beet and sweet potato into ½-inch cubes.
2. In a steamer, add 1 inch of water and bring to a boil over medium-high heat, about 2 minutes. Add cubed sweet potato and beet to the steamer basket and cover. Steam for 8–10 minutes. When done, you should be able to easily push a fork through to the center of the cubes.
3. Remove from heat and allow to cool for 5 minutes.
4. Add cubed vegetables, chickpeas, tahini, garlic, turmeric, and salt to a food processor. Puree in 30-second increments and slowly drizzle in olive oil until the hummus reaches a creamy consistency.

Cottage Cheese Fruit Bowl

A cottage cheese fruit bowl is a perfect light but tasty snack that can be prepared in under 5 minutes. This recipe includes peaches and oranges, but just about any fruit high in antioxidants can be substituted. This includes blueberries, raspberries, apples, strawberries, and blackberries.

Nutritional Information:

- Calories: 87
- Total fat: 3 g
- Total carbohydrates: 11 g
- Sugar: 8 g
- Fiber: 2 g
- Protein: 7 g
- Sodium: 199 mg

Time: 5 minutes

Serving Size: ½ cup (yields 1 serving)

Ingredients:

- ¼ cup cottage cheese
- ¼ peach, sliced
- ¼ orange, sliced

Directions:

1. Scoop cottage cheese into a small bowl or to-go container.
2. Slice fruit and lay on top. Alternatively, put cut fruit in a resealable bag for transportation and dip into cottage cheese.

Chapter 7: Meat and Poultry

When choosing meat and poultry on an anti-inflammatory diet, is it important to steer clear of processed meats, which can worsen inflammation, such as ham, hot dogs, canned meat, and lunch meats. Instead, choose lean meats, such as chicken and turkey. Meal plans can include limited amounts of red meat, primarily through low-fat content cuts of beef and pork.

Chicken

Garlic Chicken

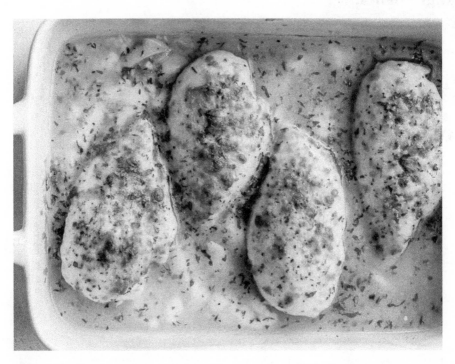

This chicken recipe packs plenty of anti-inflammatory power through its use of garlic. Not only does the garlic give the chicken great flavor, but it also contains the anti-inflammatory compound diallyl disulfide, which helps to fight back against painful and irritating inflammation.

Nutritional Information:

- Calories: 214
- Total fat: 4 g
- Total carbohydrates: 3 g
- Sugar: <1 g
- Fiber: <1 g
- Protein: 38 g
- Sodium: 479 mg

Time: 25 minutes

Serving Size: 1 chicken breast (yields 3 servings)

Ingredients:

- 3 pounds chicken breast
- 2 tablespoons garlic powder
- 1 teaspoon paprika
- ½ teaspoon salt
- ½ teaspoon ground black pepper

Directions:

1. Preheat oven to 450 degrees Fahrenheit.
2. In a small bowl, mix garlic powder, paprika, salt, and pepper.
3. Grease a baking sheet and space out the chicken breasts.
4. Spread the spice mixture evenly on top of the chicken breasts.
5. Bake for 20 minutes in the oven. Cut open to ensure there is no pink remaining before serving.

Chicken Coconut Curry

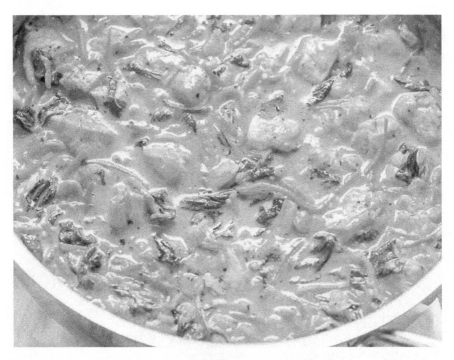

Turmeric is a common ingredient in yellow curry, and with its anti-inflammatory properties, there's no reason you have to give up curry to avoid inflammation. This chicken coconut curry takes full advantage of its ingredients' health and taste benefits to deliver a meal that is sure to impress.

Nutritional Information:

- Calories: 502
- Total fat: 40 g
- Total carbohydrates: 9 g
- Sugar: 2 g
- Fiber: 2 g
- Protein: 34 g
- Sodium: 1,415 mg

Time: 40 minutes

Serving Size: 1 chicken thigh (yields 4 servings)

Ingredients:

- 1½ pounds bone-in chicken thighs with skin
- ½ medium onion
- 1 yellow bell pepper
- 1 can (13½ ounces) coconut milk
- ½ lime
- 1 tablespoon fish sauce
- 1 tablespoon olive oil
- 1 tablespoon yellow curry paste
- 2 teaspoon turmeric
- 1 teaspoon salt
- 1 teaspoon ground black pepper

Directions:

1. Preheat oven to 375 degrees Fahrenheit.
2. Season chicken thighs with salt and pepper. Heat olive oil in an oven-proof skillet over high heat on the stovetop and then add chicken to pan skin side down.
3. Cook chicken for 8 minutes without adjusting or flipping, allowing the skin to become crispy.
4. Flip chicken, and then transfer the skillet to the oven. Bake for 20 minutes, and then remove chicken from skillet and set aside.
5. While chicken is baking, dice the onion and yellow bell pepper.
6. Remove fat and drippings from the pan. Add yellow curry paste and sauté over medium heat for about 1 minute.
7. Add diced bell pepper and onion to the skillet and cook for 5 minutes until softened. Pour in the coconut milk and turmeric.
8. Raise the heat to high and bring mixture to a boil. Then reduce heat to low and simmer until thickened, about 10 minutes.
9. Mix in fish sauce and lime juice. Add chicken thighs back into pan and coat liberally with sauce before serving.

Honey Chicken

This honey chicken recipe is quick and easy, which is perfect for a weeknight dinner. The sweetness of the honey and the slight heat of the cayenne pepper give this chicken a bold, savory flavor in no time at all.

Nutritional Information:

- Calories: 337
- Total fat: 22 g
- Total carbohydrates: 7 g
- Sugar: 6 g
- Fiber: <1 g
- Protein: 32 g
- Sodium: 446 mg

Time: 20 minutes

Serving Size: 1 chicken thigh (yields 4 servings)

Ingredients:

- 1½ pounds boneless chicken thighs with skin
- 2 tablespoons garlic, minced
- 1½ tablespoons honey
- 1 tablespoon olive oil
- 1 tablespoon soy sauce
- ½ teaspoon clove
- ½ teaspoon rosemary
- ½ teaspoon cayenne pepper

Directions:

1. In a bowl, combine garlic, honey, soy sauce, clove, rosemary, and cayenne pepper.
2. Add chicken to the bowl and coat in sauce.
3. Heat olive oil in a skillet on medium heat. Cook chicken until golden brown and no pink remains, about 8 minutes on each side.

Turmeric Lime Chicken

This turmeric lime chicken recipe helps to spice up chicken and keep things fresh and interesting. If you typically bake or grill your chicken, pan-frying is a great way to keep the chicken moist while also getting it nice and crispy on the outside. The flavors from the turmeric, lime, and parsley elevate this dish to the next level.

Nutritional Information:

- Calories: 309
- Total fat: 14 g
- Total carbohydrates: 8 g
- Sugar: 2 g
- Fiber: 3 g
- Protein: 38 g
- Sodium: 1,643 mg

Time: 50 minutes

Serving Size: 1 chicken breast (yields 3 servings)

Ingredients:

- 3 pounds chicken breasts
- 2 limes, halved
- 2 tablespoons parsley
- 2 tablespoons garlic, minced
- 2 tablespoons olive oil
- 1 tablespoon turmeric
- ¼ cup cherry tomatoes
- 2 teaspoon salt
- 2 teaspoon ground black pepper

Directions:

1. Season chicken on both sides with salt and pepper.
2. Wash parsley and chop into fine pieces.

3. In a bowl, juice limes. Add garlic and chopped parsley. Add the chicken and allow to marinate, covered at room temperature, for 30 minutes.
4. To a skillet, add olive oil and chicken. Season chicken with turmeric, and pan-fry over medium heat until done, about 8 minutes per side, depending on the thickness of the chicken breast. Check to ensure there is no pink visible after cooking.
5. Add cherry tomatoes and cook for another 3 minutes, just until softened. Plate and serve.

Pork

Maple Pork Chops

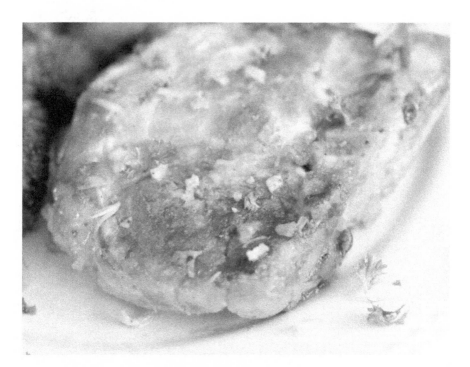

Pork is a great lean protein choice. It makes a good base for all sorts of anti-inflammatory spices and pairs nicely with a maple glaze. Best of all, this maple pork chops recipe only requires a single pan, so you can save time on both prep work and clean-up after dinner.

Nutritional Information:

- Calories: 375
- Total fat: 21 g
- Total carbohydrates: 4 g
- Sugar: 12 g
- Fiber: <1 g
- Protein: 40 g

- Sodium: 309 mg

Time: 20 minutes

Serving Size: 1 pork chop (yields 4 servings)

Ingredients:

- 2½ pounds bone-in pork chops
- 1 tablespoon pure maple syrup
- 1 tablespoon spicy brown mustard
- 1 tablespoon olive oil
- 2 teaspoon garlic, minced
- 1 teaspoon ginger, ground or grated
- ½ teaspoon pink Himalayan salt
- ½ teaspoon ground black pepper

Directions:

1. Preheat oven to 450 degrees Fahrenheit.
2. In a small bowl, add olive oil, maple syrup, and mustard. Whisk to combine.
3. Line a baking sheet with aluminum foil. Lay the pork chops out on a baking sheet.
4. Spoon the oil, maple syrup, and mustard mix onto the pork chops. Evenly spread the garlic on top. Dust with ginger, salt, and pepper.
5. Put the sheet pan in the oven and roast for 15 minutes.

Turmeric Pork Chops

Turmeric's great anti-inflammatory abilities can also be applied to pork chops. This recipe utilizes turmeric as a breading replacement to give the pork chops a crispy exterior. Pan-frying keeps the dish moist and locks in flavor.

Nutritional Information:

- Calories: 402
- Total fat: 24 g

- Total carbohydrates: 3 g
- Sugar: <1 g
- Fiber: 2 g
- Protein: 41 g
- Sodium: 1,250 mg

Time: 15 minutes

Serving Size: 1 pork chop (yields 4 servings)

Ingredients:

- 2½ pounds boneless pork chops
- 2 tablespoons olive oil
- 2 tablespoons turmeric
- 3 teaspoons paprika
- 2 teaspoons salt
- 1 teaspoon sage

Directions:

1. In a bowl, combine turmeric, paprika, salt, and sage.
2. Coat pork chops in spice mix one at a time by adding to a bowl and flipping until both sides are seasoned.
3. Heat olive oil in a skillet on medium heat. Pan-fry pork chops until spice mix is crispy, about 4 minutes on each side.

Other Meats

Sesame Meatballs

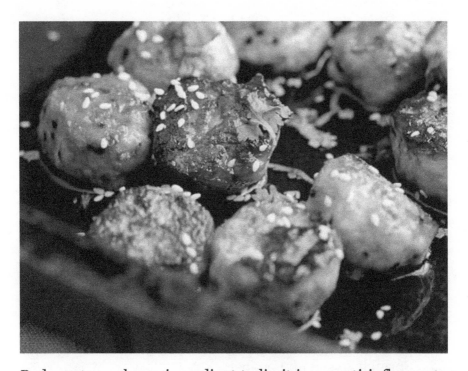

Red meat may be an ingredient to limit in an anti-inflammatory diet, but there are ways you can still incorporate it into your meals without risking inflammation. If you're using beef, choose leaner cuts of meat with lower fat content when possible, and make good use of inflammation-fighting ingredients. These sesame meatballs are a great way to include a limited amount of red meat in your meal plan.

Nutritional Information:

- Calories: 186
- Total fat: 9 g
- Total carbohydrates: 8 g
- Sugar: <1 g

- Fiber: 1 g
- Protein: 20 g
- Sodium: 481 mg

Time: 25 minutes

Serving Size: 3 meatballs (yields 4 servings)

Ingredients:

- 1 pound lean ground beef
- ¼ cup whole grain bread crumbs
- 1 egg
- 2 tablespoons parsley, finely chopped
- 1 tablespoon oregano, finely chopped
- 1 tablespoon soy sauce
- 2 teaspoons sesame oil
- 2 teaspoons ginger, ground or grated
- 1 teaspoon salt
- 1 teaspoon ground black pepper

Directions:

1. Preheat oven to 450 degrees Fahrenheit.
2. To a large bowl, add ground beef, bread crumbs, egg, parsley, oregano, soy sauce, sesame oil, and ginger. Sprinkle in salt and pepper.
3. Using a hand mixer set to low, blend ingredients until uniform. Do not overmix; you may prefer to mix by hand after using the mixer to ensure no egg or bread crumbs remain at the bottom of the bowl.
4. Grease a baking sheet. Roll the meat mixture into 12 meatballs, keeping sizes as even as possible.
5. Bake for 18–20 minutes and serve.

Ground Turkey Skillet

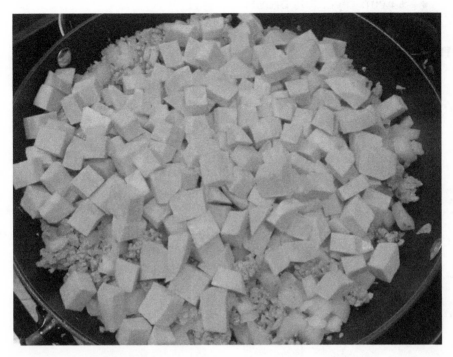

Nutritional Information:

- Calories: 243
- Total fat: 17 g
- Total carbohydrates: 9 g
- Sugar: 2 g
- Fiber: 1 g
- Protein: 15 g
- Sodium: 101 mg

Time: 30 minutes

Serving Size: 1 cup (yields 4 servings)

Ingredients:

- 1 pound ground turkey
- ½ medium yellow onion
- 1 sweet potato

- ½ yellow pepper
- ¼ cup vegetable broth
- 2 tablespoons olive oil

Directions:

1. Dice onion, yellow pepper, and sweet potato. Add olive oil to a skillet on medium heat and stir in onions and yellow peppers. Sauté until soft, about 4 minutes.
2. Add in sweet potato. Cover and cook for 5 minutes.
3. Remove onions, yellow peppers, and sweet potato from the pan and set aside, leaving behind remaining olive oil. Add ground turkey and cook until browned, about 5 minutes.
4. Return vegetables to the skillet and add in the vegetable broth. Cover and let simmer for 5 minutes.
5. Remove cover and cook for two 2 minutes before serving.

Chapter 8: Seafood

Seafood is an amazing anti-inflammatory protein option. Fish is full of healthy omega-3 fatty acids, which are both good for you and great for weight loss. Food with high-fat content can make you feel fuller faster, and as long as those fats are unsaturated (like the kind found in seafood), they are a great alternative to consuming high amounts of carbs.

Shrimp

Shrimp Scampi with Zucchini Noodles

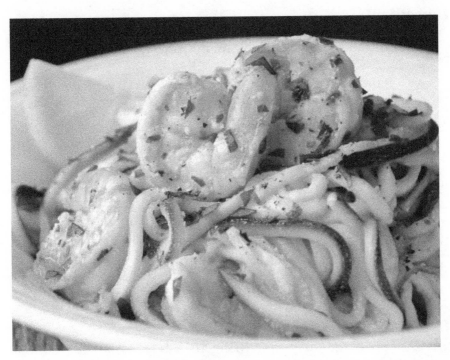

Zucchini noodles (also referred to a zoodles) are the perfect pasta replacement. High in fiber and low in calories, zucchini is both anti-inflammatory and an overall healthier choice than spaghetti or angel hair pasta. Complement your zoodles with shrimp cooked in a lemon butter sauce, and this shrimp scampi recipe may even surpass the real deal.

Nutritional Information:

- Calories: 183
- Total fat: 15 g
- Total carbohydrates: 7 g
- Sugar: 2 g
- Fiber: 2 g
- Protein: 8 g
- Sodium: 774 mg

Time: 20 minutes

Serving Size: 1 cup (yields 4 servings)

Ingredients:

- 1 pound shrimp, peeled and deveined
- 2 cups spiralized zucchini
- 1 lemon
- ½ cup vegetable broth
- 4 tablespoons garlic, minced
- 4 tablespoons olive oil
- 2 tablespoons parsley, finely chopped
- 1 teaspoon pink Himalayan salt
- ¼ teaspoon black pepper
- ¼ teaspoon paprika

Directions:

1. Pour oil into a large skillet over medium heat. Add garlic and sauté until fragrant, about 1 minute. Be sure to continually stir the garlic to avoid burning.
2. Add in vegetable broth, pink Himalayan salt, black pepper, and paprika. Bring to a boil, about 4 minutes, and then reduce heat to low. Simmer for 5 minutes.

3. Add shrimp to the skillet and cook until pink on both sides, about 3 minutes. Sprinkle in parsley, and squeeze the juice from the lemon over the shrimp.
4. Stir in zucchini noodles and coat well in sauce. Cook for 2 minutes until zucchini has softened, and serve.

Sesame Shrimp Stir-Fry

Shrimp is high in healthy fats, and choosing seafood meals over other proteins can yield a significant reduction in inflammation. This sesame shrimp stir-fry combines all the best aspects of Chinese take-out without any of the inflammation.

Nutritional Information:

- Calories: 199
- Total fat: 11 g
- Total carbohydrates: 17 g
- Sugar: 4 g
- Fiber: 2 g
- Protein: 10 g
- Sodium: 1,176 mg

Time: 20 minutes

Serving Size: ½ cup (yields 4 servings)

Ingredients:

- 1 pound shrimp, peeled and deveined
- 1 yellow onion
- 1 red bell pepper
- ½ cup button mushrooms
- ¼ cup soy sauce
- 2 tablespoons garlic, minced
- 2 tablespoons honey
- 2 tablespoons sesame seeds
- 2 tablespoons olive oil
- 2 teaspoons sesame oil

Directions:

1. Cut the onion and mushrooms into thin slices. Dice red bell pepper.
2. In a skillet over medium heat, add 1 tablespoon olive oil and shrimp. Stir-fry until pink on both sides, about 3 minutes. Remove shrimp from heat and set aside.
3. Pour the remaining 1 tablespoon olive oil into the skillet and add onions, peppers, and mushrooms. Stir-fry until tender, about 5 minutes.
4. Add garlic and cook for 1 minute.
5. In a bowl, mix together soy sauce, honey, sesame seeds, and sesame oil.
6. Pour the sauce into the skillet, and return shrimp to the pan. Cook for 2 minutes, just until the sauce has thickened.

Salmon

Honey Mustard Salmon

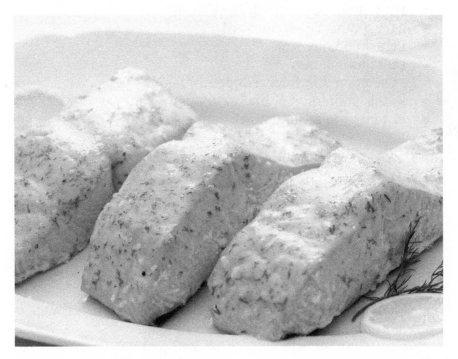

Honey mustard's sweetness and tanginess is great with salmon, but normal honey mustard is very high in sugar. Skip the prepackaged bottles and whip up quick homemade honey mustard for all the flavor and none of the refined sugars.

Nutritional Information:

- Calories: 518
- Total fat: 32 g
- Total carbohydrates: 5 g
- Sugar: 4 g
- Fiber: <1 g
- Protein: 50 g
- Sodium: 273 mg

Time: 15 minutes

Serving Size: 1 salmon fillet (yields 2 servings)

Ingredients:

- 1½ pounds salmon fillets, skin-on
- 2 teaspoons Dijon mustard
- 1 teaspoon olive oil
- 1 teaspoon honey
- 1 teaspoon dill, finely chopped
- ½ teaspoon thyme, finely chopped
- ½ teaspoon ground black pepper

Directions:

1. Preheat oven to 425 degrees Fahrenheit.
2. In a bowl, add mustard, olive oil, honey, dill, thyme, and black pepper. Whisk together to combine into honey mustard mixture.
3. Line a baking sheet with aluminum foil. Lay salmon out skin side down on the baking sheet and top with honey mustard mixture.
4. Bake in the oven for about 8 minutes until salmon is flaky and easily separable from its skin.

Lemon-Pepper Turmeric Salmon

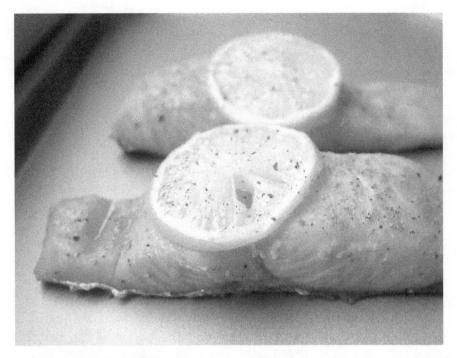

Turmeric can be incorporated into salmon recipes as a potent anti-inflammatory ingredient. Combined with the healthy fats of salmon, this lemon-pepper turmeric salmon recipe packs plenty of inflammation-fighting punch.

Nutritional Information:

- Calories: 503
- Total fat: 28 g
- Total carbohydrates: 10 g
- Sugar: 1 g
- Fiber: 2 g
- Protein: 51 g
- Sodium: 140 mg

Time: 1 hour 15 minutes

Serving Size: 1 salmon fillet (yields 2 servings)

Ingredients:

- 1½ pounds salmon fillets, skin-on
- 1 lemon
- 1 teaspoon ground black pepper
- 1 teaspoon thyme, finely chopped
- 1 teaspoon rosemary, finely chopped
- ½ teaspoon honey
- ½ teaspoon turmeric

Directions:

1. In a small bowl, squeeze the juice from the lemon. Mix in black pepper, thyme, rosemary, honey, and turmeric.
2. Marinate salmon by placing fillets in a large resealable bag and pouring lemon marinade into the bag. Seal and refrigerate for 1 hour.
3. Preheat oven to 400 degrees Fahrenheit.
4. Line a baking sheet with aluminum foil and transfer salmon from the fridge to the baking sheet, placing the fillets skin side up. Do not throw out the marinade bag.
5. Bake for 6 minutes. Remove from oven and flip salmon over so that the fillets are skin side down. Spoon 2 tablespoons of the marinade on top.
6. Return the salmon to the oven and bake for another 6 minutes until salmon is flaky.

Lemon Garlic Salmon

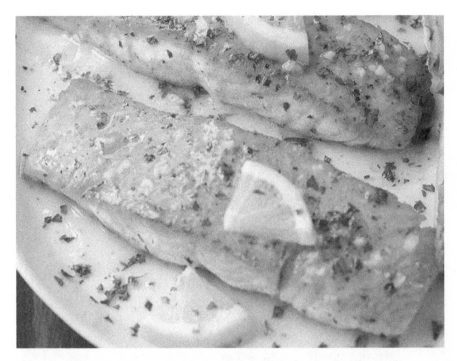

Lemon and garlic go great with fish, and both have good antioxidant content and anti-inflammatory abilities. Take advantage of this by pairing them with salmon, which is anti-inflammatory and has plenty of healthy fats to keep you full and fit.

Nutritional Information:

- Calories: 606
- Total fat: 39 g
- Total carbohydrates: 11 g
- Sugar: 3 g
- Fiber: 4 g
- Protein: 54 g
- Sodium: 258 mg

Time: 15 minutes

Serving Size: 1 salmon fillet (yields 4 servings)

Ingredients:

- 3 pounds salmon fillets, skin-on
- 1½ pounds asparagus
- 2 lemons
- 3 tablespoons garlic, minced
- 3 tablespoons olive oil
- 1 tablespoon dill, chopped
- 1 teaspoon pink Himalayan salt
- ½ teaspoon ground black pepper

Directions:

1. Turn on the broiler to preheat.
2. Line a baking sheet with aluminum foil and lay out salmon fillets skin side down.
3. Rinse asparagus and arrange on the baking sheet next to the salmon without overlapping. Sprinkle salmon and asparagus with salt and pepper, and season salmon with chopped dill.
4. Cut one lemon in half and juice into a small bowl. With a zester or grater, add about 1 tablespoon of zest to the lemon juice. Mix with olive oil and garlic. Drizzle lemon mixture over the asparagus and salmon.
5. Cut the other lemon into thin slices and spread across salmon fillets and asparagus.
6. Broil for 8–10 minutes or until salmon is flaky and separates easily from its skin.

Tuna

Tuna Salad Avocado Boats

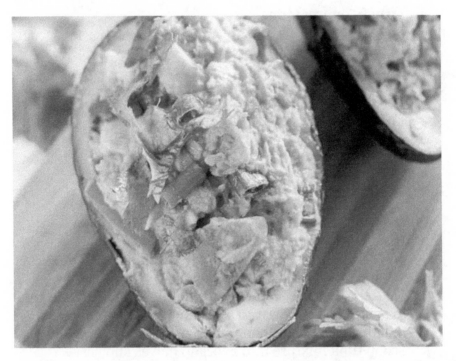

Combine the blood pressure and immune system benefits of tuna and the vitamins and healthy fats of avocados with these tuna salad avocado boats. Quick to make and easy to eat on-the-go or while multitasking, this recipe is wonderful for busy weekdays.

Nutritional Information:

- Calories: 286
- Total fat: 15 g
- Total carbohydrates: 14 g
- Sugar: 4 g
- Fiber: 8 g
- Protein: 25 g
- Sodium: 653 mg

Time: 10 minutes

Serving Size: 1 avocado boat (yields 2 servings)

Ingredients:

- 1 can (5 ounces) tuna
- 1 avocado
- ¼ red onion
- ¼ cup shredded carrots
- 2 tablespoons nonfat Greek yogurt
- 4 teaspoons apple cider vinegar
- 1 teaspoon curry powder
- 1 teaspoon paprika
- ½ teaspoon salt

Directions:

1. Dice onion and carrots.
2. In a bowl, combine yogurt, apple cider vinegar, curry powder, paprika, and salt. Stir in diced onion and carrots.
3. Add tuna and mix until well coated.
4. Take the avocado and cut it in half lengthwise, rotating it to avoid the pit. Twist to separate into halves and remove the pit with a large spoon.
5. Scoop tuna mixture into avocado halves and serve.

Sundried-Tomato Tuna Flatbread

If you're looking for an easy and filling meal, look no further than this sundried-tomato tuna flatbread. The sundried tomato gives the tuna great flavor, and the whole meal can be made in just 10 minutes, no cooking required.

Nutritional Information:

- Calories: 318
- Total fat: 9 g
- Total carbohydrates: 35 g
- Sugar: 5 g
- Fiber: 8 g
- Protein: 29 g
- Sodium: 439 mg

Time: 10 minutes

Serving Size: ½ flatbread (yields 2 servings)

Ingredients:

- 1 can (5 ounces) tuna
- 1 whole wheat flatbread
- ½ avocado
- ½ lemon
- ½ cup spinach
- ¼ cup sundried tomatoes
- ½ teaspoon coriander

Directions:

1. Wash and chop spinach and coriander. Dice sundried tomatoes.
2. Cut avocado in half lengthwise, rotating as you cut to avoid the pit, and twist the two halves apart. Scoop out and discard the pit, and scoop remaining avocado onto flatbread. Mash with a fork.
3. Spread tuna on top of the flatbread. Top with spinach, sundried tomatoes, coriander, and lemon juice.

Chapter 9: Vegetarian Recipes

Whether you are looking to cut meat out of your diet completely or only looking for more variety in your meals, vegetarian recipes can be a great option when it comes to anti-inflammatory cooking. Reducing how often you eat meat, even without being strictly vegetarian or vegan, can benefit your heart health and reduce the risk of cardiovascular disease. However, if you're not committed to going meatless, these vegetarian dishes can still satisfy as great meal options.

Lunches

Ginger Carrot Soup

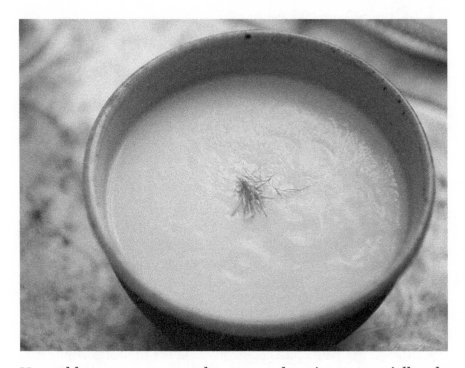

Vegetable soups are great hearty meal options, especially when the weather takes a turn for the worse and the warm soup combats the harsh cold outside. On these days, enjoy a nice relaxing bowl of soup with added anti-inflammatory benefits.

Nutritional Information:

- Calories: 91
- Total fat: 6 g
- Total carbohydrates: 11 g
- Sugar: 3 g
- Fiber: 3 g
- Protein: 2 g
- Sodium: 84 mg

Time: 45 minutes

Serving Size: 1 cup (yields 8 servings)

Ingredients:

- 3 cups carrots
- 3 cups low sodium vegetable broth
- 1 can (14.5 ounces) light coconut milk
- 2 leeks
- 1 butternut squash
- 2 tablespoons garlic, minced
- 1 tablespoon ginger, ground or grated
- 1 tablespoon turmeric
- 1 tablespoon olive oil
- 1 teaspoon ground black pepper

Directions:

1. Slice off the top and bottom ends of the butternut squash with a large knife. Using a vegetable peeler, peel until the darker orange flesh is visible. Stand the squash up vertically on the cutting board, and slice in half. Use a spoon to remove seeds.
2. Chop carrots, leeks, and squash into ¼-inch size chunks.
3. In a large saucepan, heat olive oil on medium-high. Add the carrots, squash, and leeks. Sauté until softened, about 3 minutes.
4. Add garlic, ginger, turmeric, and black pepper. Sauté for another 2 minutes.
5. Pour in coconut milk and vegetable broth. Bring to a boil over high heat, about 6 minutes. Then reduce heat to medium-low, cover the saucepan, and leave to simmer for 20 minutes.
6. After simmering, remove soup from heat and let cool for 10 minutes to avoid putting hot liquids in the blender. Transfer to a blender and blend on low in 30-second intervals for about 2 minutes or until creamy. Return to saucepan and heat through, about 4 minutes, and serve once hot.

Kiwi and Pineapple Smoothie

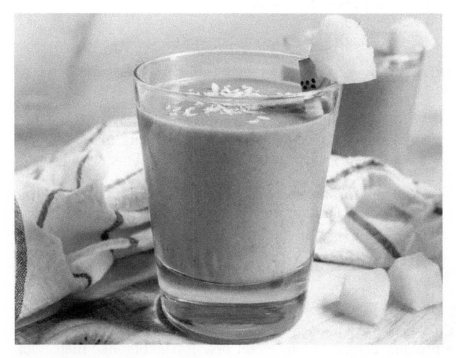

Nutritional Information:

- Calories: 124
- Total fat: 2 g
- Total carbohydrates: 26 g
- Sugar: 14 g
- Fiber: 7 g
- Protein: 5 g
- Sodium: 67 mg

Time: 5 minutes

Serving Size: 8 ounces (yields 2 servings)

Ingredients:

- 1 cup pineapple, chunked, frozen or chilled
- 2 kiwis
- 1 cup spinach, frozen

- 1 cup water
- 2 teaspoons chia seeds
- 1 teaspoon turmeric
- 1 teaspoon ginger, ground or grated

Directions:

1. Slice ends off the kiwis and scoop out the fruit into a blender. Add pineapple chunks and spinach.
2. Blend for 30 seconds to break ingredients apart.
3. Add chia seeds, turmeric, and ginger. Pour in half of the water.
4. Blend for 20 seconds, add the remaining water, and blend for another 20 seconds or until desired consistency is reached.

Shawarma Dip

Chickpeas are a high-protein food often used in place of meat as a protein. They also have great health benefits, like their high-fiber content, which aids digestion, and their ability to reduce inflammation. This meat-free shawarma dip recipe is a great addition to any vegetarian meal plan. It can be eaten as is or served with crunchy kale chips or sliced vegetables for dipping.

Nutritional Information:

- Calories: 207
- Total fat: 13 g
- Total carbohydrates: 19 g
- Sugar: 4 g
- Fiber: 5 g
- Protein: 6 g
- Sodium: 450 mg

Time: 15 minutes

Serving Size: ½ cup (yields 4 servings)

Ingredients:

- 1 can (15 ounces) chickpeas
- ½ cup tahini
- ¼ red onion
- 1 lemon
- ½ cup parsley, finely chopped
- ¼ cup cherry tomatoes
- 2 tablespoons garlic
- 2 tablespoons olive oil
- 1 teaspoon paprika
- ½ teaspoon salt
- ½ teaspoon dill, finely chopped

Directions:

1. Begin by making the hummus base. In a microwave-safe bowl, combine the can of chickpeas and garlic. Do not drain chickpeas. Microwave on high for 5 minutes.
2. Allow chickpeas to cool for 1 minute and then transfer to a blender. Squeeze the juice from ½ lemon into the blender. Add tahini, salt, and olive oil. Blend until smooth, about 2 minutes.
3. Wash and halve cherry tomatoes. Dice red onion.
4. In a large container or on a serving platter, spread hummus base and top with cherry tomatoes, red onion, parsley, dill, and the juice of ½ lemon. Sprinkle paprika on top and serve.

Dinners

Vegetable Shepherd's Pie

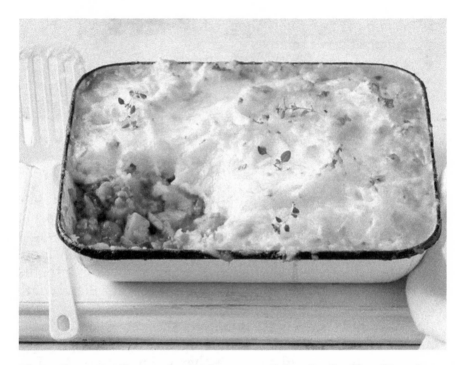

Though typically made with ground beef, shepherd's pie can easily be altered to a vegetarian recipe. Ditch the meat and try this satisfying dinner full of healthy veggies and topped with perfectly golden-brown mashed potatoes.

Nutritional Information:

- Calories: 336
- Total fat: 10 g
- Total carbohydrates: 54 g
- Sugar: 9 g
- Fiber: 8 g
- Protein: 8 g
- Sodium: 104 mg

Time: 40 minutes

Serving Size: 1 cup (yields 6 servings)

Ingredients:

- 4 red potatoes
- 2 cups low sodium vegetable broth
- 2 cups carrots, shredded
- 2 cups peas
- 1 cup button mushrooms
- ¼ cup sour cream
- ½ yellow onion, diced
- 4 tablespoons olive oil
- 2 tablespoons tomato paste
- 2 tablespoons garlic

Directions:

1. Peel potatoes and cut into quarters. In a pot, add 2 cups of salted water and bring to a boil, about 4 minutes. Cook for 15 minutes or until tender enough to be easily pierced with a fork.
2. Drain water from the pot and remove from heat. Mash potatoes and stir in sour cream and 2 tablespoons oil.
3. Preheat oven to 350 degrees Fahrenheit.
4. In an oven-safe pot, add the remainder of the olive oil and warm on medium heat. Add mushrooms, carrots, onions, and garlic. Sauté to soften, about 4 minutes.
5. Stir in tomato paste and broth. Allow it to thicken over low heat for about 3 minutes.
6. Mix in peas and spread potatoes on top as an even layer. Transfer to oven and bake for 15 minutes.

Stuffed Sweet Potatoes

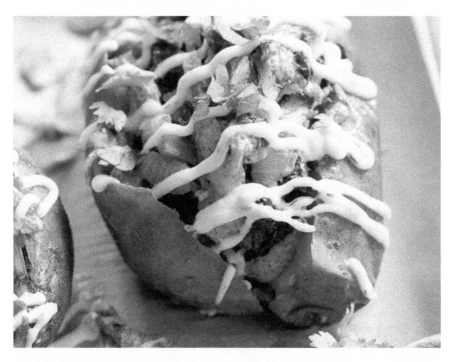

Stuffed sweet potatoes are a simple and delicious meal that can be customized with a variety of fillings. This recipe uses black beans and sundried tomatoes, but you can also try a mini kale salad, maple-glazed walnuts, or a vegetarian chili for some variation.

Nutritional Information:

- Calories: 267
- Total fat: 8 g
- Total carbohydrates: 42 g
- Sugar: 8 g
- Fiber: 11 g
- Protein: 9 g
- Sodium: 1,031 mg

Time: 55 minutes

Serving Size: 1 sweet potato (yields 4 servings)

Ingredients:

- 4 sweet potatoes
- 1 can (15 ounces) black beans
- ½ white onion, minced
- ¼ cup sundried tomatoes, halved
- 2 tablespoons olive oil
- 1 tablespoon garlic
- 1 teaspoon clove
- 1 teaspoon salt

Directions:

1. Preheat oven to 350 degrees Fahrenheit.
2. Line a baking sheet with aluminum foil and lay sweet potatoes on top. Drizzle 1 tablespoon olive oil over sweet potatoes and bake for 45 minutes.
3. Add 1 tablespoon olive oil to a skillet and sauté onion over medium heat for 4 minutes. Add garlic and cook for another 2 minutes, stirring frequently.
4. Add sundried tomatoes and black beans to onions and garlic and cook until warmed, about 2 minutes.
5. Make a long lengthwise cut in the sweet potatoes and pull apart to lay flat. Spoon onions, garlic, beans, and tomatoes on top. Sprinkle with clove and salt and serve.

Sweet Potato and Broccoli Casserole

Casseroles are great for feeding large groups of people or for whipping up on a weekend to enjoy over the course of the week. This sweet potato and broccoli casserole features a basil and parsley pesto that ties the ingredients together for a dish you won't mind eating as leftovers for a few days.

Nutritional Information:

- Calories: 133

- Total fat: 11 g
- Total carbohydrates: 8 g
- Sugar: 2 g
- Fiber: 2 g
- Protein: 3 g
- Sodium: 825 mg

Time: 50 minutes

Serving Size: 1 cup (yields 6 servings)

Ingredients:

- 2 cups broccoli, chopped
- 1 sweet potato
- ⅓ cup vegetable broth
- 2½ cups basil
- ¼ cup parsley
- 2 tablespoons pine nuts
- 2 tablespoons olive oil
- 1 tablespoon garlic
- 2 teaspoons salt
- 2 teaspoons ground black pepper

Directions:

1. Preheat oven to 400 degrees Fahrenheit.
2. Cut off the ends of the sweet potato and peel. Cut the sweet potato into chunks of roughly one inch.
3. Add sweet potato to a food processor and pulse until riced, about 2 minutes. Remove riced sweet potato and set aside.
4. Add basil, parsley, pine nuts, olive oil, and garlic to the food processor. Season with salt and pepper. Pulse for 1 minute or until well blended.
5. Spread a thin layer of about half of the pesto on the bottom of a casserole dish. Add a layer of sweet potato rice, and then the broccoli. Top with the remainder of the sweet potato rice and the remaining pesto.

6. Pour vegetable broth evenly over the casserole.
7. Cover the casserole dish in aluminum foil. Bake for 40 minutes.

Chapter 10: Desserts

Most standard desserts are off-limits on an anti-inflammatory diet due to their high sugar and refined grain content. You won't be able to buy a box of brownie mix or pick up a cake at the store. However, this does not mean you can no longer enjoy a treat after dinner; in fact, it doesn't even mean that brownies and cakes are off the table if they are made with the right ingredients. Ingredient restrictions just mean anti-inflammatory dessert recipes tend to get creative, which can lead to surprisingly tasty results.

Frozen Desserts

Berry Ice Pops

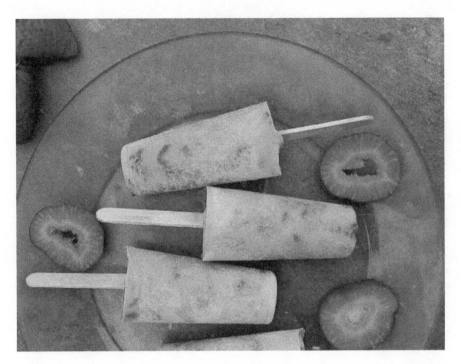

These berry ice pops boast an incredibly simple recipe, requiring only four ingredients to prepare a quick treat for any season. For the classic ice-pop shape, use popsicle molds, but paper cups also work well in a pinch.

Nutritional Information:

- Calories: 74
- Total fat: <1 g
- Total carbohydrates: 10 g
- Sugar: 10 g
- Fiber: <1 g
- Protein: 7 g
- Sodium: 92 mg

Time: 10 minutes/overnight

Serving Size: 1 ice pop (yields 6 servings)

Ingredients:

- 3 cups nonfat yogurt
- 1 cup strawberries, stems removed
- 1 tablespoon almonds
- ¼ lemon

Directions:

1. In a blender, add strawberries and almonds. Blend until broken down into a slushy-like consistency, about 1 minute.
2. Scoop in yogurt and add lemon juice. Blend to combine, about 20–30 seconds.
3. Pour mixture into six ice pop molds or a freezer-safe container. Place a popsicle stick inside each.
4. Freeze overnight.

Chocolate-Dipped Frozen Bananas

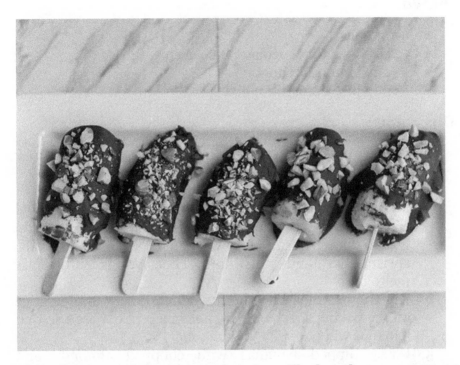

Though it is much less sweet than its milk chocolate counterpart, dark chocolate boasts a variety of health benefits, including positive effects on blood pressure, cholesterol, and inflammation. These banana pops pair dark chocolate with the salty taste and crunchy texture of almonds and pistachios for a sweet treat.

Nutritional Information:

- Calories: 248
- Total fat: 12 g
- Total carbohydrates: 32 g
- Sugar: 22 g
- Fiber: 4 g
- Protein: 3 g
- Sodium: 12 mg

Time: 10 minutes/overnight

Serving Size: 1 banana pop (yields 9 servings)

Ingredients:

- 3 bananas
- 12 ounces dark chocolate, 85% cocoa or higher
- ¼ cup almonds, chopped
- ¼ cup pistachios, chopped

Directions:

1. Peel bananas and cut into thirds. Stick a popsicle stick into each, about ¾ of the way through the banana.
2. Line a baking sheet with parchment paper.
3. Melt dark chocolate in a double boiler. Alternatively, you can melt the chocolate in the microwave, but be careful not to let it burn. Microwave in 15-second intervals, stirring frequently, just until chocolate is sufficiently melted.
4. Dip the bananas into the melted chocolate and arrange on the baking sheet with enough space in between so that bananas will not stick to each other.
5. Cover dipped bananas with chopped almonds and pistachios and allow to set in the freezer. For best results, freeze overnight.

Chocolate Parfait

Thankfully, lowering the amount of refined sugar in your diet doesn't mean you have to give up chocolate. This chocolate parfait recipe uses cocoa powder and natural sweeteners to make a parfait so good it tastes just like the real deal.

Nutritional Information:

- Calories: 89
- Total fat: 2 g
- Total carbohydrates: 12 g
- Sugar: 11 g

- Fiber: 1 g
- Protein: 5 g
- Sodium: 19 mg

Time: 5 minutes

Serving Size: 1 parfait (yields 4 servings)

Ingredients:

- 1 cup nonfat Greek yogurt
- 1 cup blueberries
- ½ cup raspberries
- ½ cup strawberries, sliced
- 2 tablespoons walnuts
- 1 teaspoon vanilla extract
- 1 teaspoon honey
- ½ teaspoon cocoa powder
- ½ teaspoon cinnamon

Directions:

1. Add yogurt, cocoa powder, honey, and vanilla extract to a bowl. Mix until uniform.
2. Scoop 2 tablespoons of the yogurt mix into four serving glasses. Top with blueberries, raspberries, walnuts, and cinnamon.
3. If desired, leave in the freezer for 5 minutes to chill.

Pudding

Chocolate Cherry Pudding

The combination of chocolate and cherries is one that never disappoints. Cherries are a source of potent antioxidants and fit right in with any anti-inflammatory diet. This recipe for chocolate cherry pudding keeps things nice and simple for delicious results.

Nutritional Information:

- Calories: 109
- Total fat: 2 g
- Total carbohydrates: 21 g
- Sugar: 15 g
- Fiber: 3 g
- Protein: 2 g
- Sodium: 392 mg

Time: 15 minutes

Serving Size: ½ cup (yields 4 servings)

Ingredients:

- 1½ cup almond milk
- ½ cup cherries
- ¼ cup chia seeds
- 3 tablespoons cacao powder
- 2 tablespoons honey
- 1 teaspoon pink Himalayan salt

Directions:

1. Wash and cut cherries into fourths, discarding pits and stems.

2. In a bowl, mix together almond milk, chia seeds, cacao, and honey. Separate evenly into four glasses and top with cherries. Sprinkle with Himalayan salt.
3. Chill in the freezer for 10 minutes before serving.

Cakes and Brownies

Pineapple Upside-Down Cake

Cutting down on refined grains doesn't have to mean giving up cake. Instead, get creative with an old classic with this pineapple upside-down cake recipe and enjoy the anti-inflammatory benefits of pineapple in a dessert you can feel great about eating.

Nutritional Information:

- Calories: 200
- Total fat: 13 g
- Total carbohydrates: 17 g
- Sugar: 14 g
- Fiber: 2 g
- Protein: 5 g
- Sodium: 19 mg

Time: 1 hour

Serving Size: 1 slice (yields 8 servings)

Ingredients:

- 1 cup almond flour
- ½ cup cherries
- 3 pineapple slices (½ inch thick)
- 2 eggs
- 5 tablespoons honey

- 3 tablespoons avocado oil
- 1 teaspoon vanilla extract
- ½ teaspoon baking powder

Directions:

1. Preheat oven to 350 degrees Fahrenheit.
2. Remove the core from the pineapple slices and peel. Leave one as a solid ring shape, and cut the other two into halves.
3. In a round cake pan or cast-iron skillet, spread 2 tablespoons of honey across the bottom in an even layer. Lay a pineapple ring in the center and arrange the four halves around it, with the rounded sides facing out toward the edges of the pan. Fill in the gaps with cherries.
4. Bake the pineapple and cherries in the oven for 15 minutes.
5. While the fruit is baking, crack the eggs into a bowl and beat until uniform. Add almond flour, baking powder, avocado oil, and the remaining 3 tablespoons of honey. Mix well to form a batter.
6. Pour batter into the pan over the fruit and return to the oven for 30–35 minutes.
7. When finished cooking, let cool for 10 minutes before attempting to flip. Carefully slide a butter knife around the edges of the cake to separate it from the sides of the pan or skillet. Cover the pan with a large plate, flip over, and serve.

Avocado Brownies

The idea of avocado brownies may sound a bit like the product of a desperate parent trying to hide healthy ingredients in dessert, but considering how good these brownies are, it's hard to believe they're good for you. They also pack plenty of anti-inflammatory power from the avocados and cocoa powder.

Nutritional Information:

- Calories: 57
- Total fat: 3 g
- Total carbohydrates: 5 g
- Sugar: 3 g
- Fiber: 1 g
- Protein: 2 g
- Sodium: 40 mg

Time: 30 minutes

Serving Size: 1 brownie (yields 16 servings)

Ingredients:

- 1 avocado
- 3 eggs
- ½ cup coconut flour
- ½ cup applesauce, unsweetened
- ½ cup maple syrup
- ½ cup Dutch-processed cocoa powder, unsweetened
- ¼ cup walnuts
- 1 teaspoon baking soda
- 1 teaspoon vanilla extract
- ¼ teaspoon pink Himalayan salt

Directions:

1. Preheat oven to 350 degrees Fahrenheit.
2. Slice avocado in half lengthwise, rotating to avoid the pit, and pull halves apart. Remove and discard the pit, and scoop avocado into a blender.
3. Add applesauce, vanilla, maple syrup, and walnuts. Blend until ingredients are mixed and walnuts are crushed, about 1 minute.
4. Transfer to a large mixing bowl and add coconut flour, cocoa powder, baking soda, and salt. Stir until no traces of coconut flour remain.

5. Grease a baking dish and pour in the batter. Bake in the oven for 20–22 minutes. Let cool before dividing into 16 brownies.

Chapter 11: 7 Day Meal Plan

With so many recipes, it can be difficult to know where to begin. This meal plan made up of the recipes contained in this cookbook can help guide you toward having a successful first week on the anti-inflammatory diet and experiencing results right away. Each day includes breakfast, lunch, a snack, and dinner, with some also including dinner sides or, on occasion, dessert. Meal plans can be a crucial element in sticking to a new diet, as well as aiding in time management by laying out everything you need to grab at the grocery store for the week and cutting out the guesswork that comes with unfamiliar recipes. This one-week guide lets you cook with confidence as you take the first steps toward a life free of inflammation.

Day 1

Breakfast — ancient grains breakfast bowl

Lunch — avocado salad

Snack — cottage cheese fruit bowl

Dinner — garlic chicken

Day 2

Breakfast — pitaya smoothie

Lunch — tuna salad avocado boats

Snack — almond and blueberry yogurt

Dinner — turmeric pork chops

Side — roasted radishes

Dessert — berry ice pops

Day 3

Breakfast — turmeric cinnamon oatmeal

Lunch — sesame shrimp stir-fry

Snack — matcha smoothie

Dinner — sweet potato and broccoli casserole

Day 4

Breakfast — sweet maple rice porridge

Lunch — sundried-tomato tuna flatbread

Snack — strawberry Greek yogurt

Dinner — honey chicken

Side — caramelized butternut squash

Day 5

Breakfast — spinach and tomato omelet

Lunch — ginger carrot soup

Snack — sweet potato and beet hummus

Dinner — honey mustard salmon

Day 6

Breakfast — strawberry almond milk smoothie

Lunch — kale and berry salad

Dressing — turmeric dressing

Snack — kiwi and pineapple smoothie

Dinner — stuffed sweet potato

Dessert — avocado brownies

Day 7

Breakfast — ancient grains breakfast bowl

Lunch — lemon garlic salmon

Snack — shawarma dip

Dinner — ground turkey skillet

Side — zucchini rice

Conclusion

An anti-inflammatory diet can help you prevent further injury to your body and heal from the effects of years of eating inflammatory foods. It is never too late to start eating healthy, and there is no better way to do so than to use this cookbook as a guide to cutting out harmful foods in favor of improved nutrition. The recipes included in the meal plan above and the rest of the book are the first steps toward freeing yourself from the constraints of inflammatory pain and swelling. In no time at all, you can begin seeing results in the form of less discomfort and improved motion in swollen joints. Additionally, following these recipes can help prevent the development of related health conditions, allowing you to live a healthier, happier life. Utilize these recipes in your daily meals, alongside other lifestyle adjustments, for a new and improved state of living.

Benefits of Following the Anti-Inflammatory Diet

Many benefits of ditching inflammatory ingredients have been discussed previously, but to summarize the wide variety of benefits, they can be categorized as reducing symptoms and decreasing health risks. Using anti-inflammatory ingredients in food helps you manage inflammation and keep pain at bay. It also helps you avoid developing other health conditions or improve those that have already developed.

Reduced Symptoms

The anti-inflammatory diet cuts out foods that produce free radicals in your body and lead to inflammation. Because of this, you will experience much less severe inflammation if it occurs at all. When you are not constantly eating meals full of sugar, refined carbs, and processed meats, your body is able to break down food in a way that does not trigger inflammatory responses. The added antioxidants, vitamins, and minerals from inflammation-fighting foods mean that even if you inadvertently eat food that would normally cause your tissues to become inflamed, their effects can be minimized by the anti-inflammatory benefits of the diet. Really committing yourself to eating right will allow you to take control of your symptoms and keep them from impeding upon your life.

Decreased Health Risks

Reducing inflammation has the secondary effect of lowering your risk for developing any related health conditions. Heart, bowel, and thyroid conditions are all linked to inflammation, and your risk of contracting these disorders is drastically decreased by taking measures to target their main cause of inflammation. Inflammatory arthritis can also be held at bay, saving you years of pain and discomfort and allowing you to maintain an active lifestyle.

In addition, eating healthier itself benefits your body and can give you more energy while lowering your risk for blood clots, high cholesterol, and weight gain. Eliminating unhealthy fats, sugars, and grains improves your overall health alongside decreasing inflammation.

Other Steps to Reduce Inflammation

While changing your diet is one of the most important ways to manage inflammation at its source, there are other methods you can use to ease the related symptoms. Adding more exercise into your day can help relieve pain and prevent inflammation from building up. If inflammation strikes, medications can be used to counteract the pain, though they should be used sparingly and only when necessary. These steps, combined with sticking to an anti-inflammatory diet, can supplement pain management strategies and help you overcome especially difficult inflammation flare-ups. Consider adding them as needed to combat pain spikes and reinforce healthy behaviors.

Exercise

Physical activity is known to help when it comes to weight loss, fitness, and muscle strength, but it can also help reduce inflammation. Exercise encourages your immune system into proper functionality and leads to decreases in inflammation. The physical activity does not have to be strenuous; in fact, even taking a brisk walk can produce positive effects on the body's immune system. Exercise is best used as a preventative measure, so 20–30 minutes of light activity every day is recommended. Frequent and consistent exercise patterns give your immune system the boost it needs to function properly and limit unnecessary cases of inflammation.

Still, it's important not to overdo it with exercise. It is best practiced in moderation to give yourself time to recover in between workouts and avoid overworking muscles. Too much strain placed on your body can lead to pain in the muscles and severe shortness of breath. Doing too much exercise is not necessary to reap the anti-inflammatory benefits. Additionally, overexerting yourself can make you less likely to stick to an exercise plan the next day. Getting in a light physical activity each day is better for your body than exhausting yourself one day and skipping out on exercise the next.

Medication

Medication for inflammation should be restricted to only necessary use, and you should involve your doctor in any decisions you make, even if it is only over-the-counter medications. Your doctor may prescribe you drugs to combat inflammation or to help manage pain. Most over-the-counter anti-inflammatory medications are referred to as nonsteroidal anti-inflammatory drugs (NSAIDs). These include ibuprofen, aspirin, and naproxen. NSAIDs can lessen the pain when inflammation occurs and reduce swelling and redness. Before taking any medication, research the side effects and know the risks.

Keep in mind that medications generally treat the symptoms of the issue but not the causes. They should be used in conjunction with exercise and diet, which help your body's immune system regulate itself.

Did You Enjoyed Reading This Cookbook?

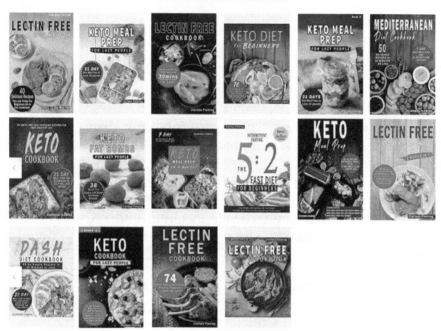

Click Here To Check Other Books By Clarissa Fleming

https://www.amazon.com/kindle-dbs/entity/author/B07H7L2Z3L

CPSIA information can be obtained
at www.ICGtesting.com
Printed in the USA
LVHW091359171219
640790LV00001B/11/P